Medical Toxicology: Antidotes and Anecdotes

Steven M. Marcus, MD

Medical Toxicology:
Antidotes and Anecdotes

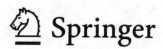 Springer

Steven M. Marcus, MD
New Jersey Medical School
School of Biomedical and Health Sciences
Rutgers, State University of New Jersey
Newark, NJ, USA

ISBN 978-3-319-84548-7   ISBN 978-3-319-51029-3   (eBook)
DOI 10.1007/978-3-319-51029-3

Printed on acid-free paper

This Springer imprint is published by Springer Nature
The registered company is Springer International Publishing AG
The registered company address is: Gewerbestrasse 11, 6330 Cham, Switzerland

Preface

Every child has a hero or two growing up. Heroes can be real people or fictional ones. They help one develop specific interests and guide the growing individual, hopefully correctly, into a chosen field. I had perhaps more than my share, but each played an important, indelible role in my development.

I grew up in Brooklyn in the 1940s and 1950s. Like many a Brooklyn boy, I had my heroes. My first was Pee Wee Reese, the Brooklyn Dodger shortstop. I remember worshipping him when I would make my almost religious-like pilgrimage to the cathedral, Ebbets Field. The Dodgers had an uncanny ability to make it just so far, only to suffer crushing defeat before achieving greatness. All Dodger fans learned to accept what we received, hoping to get more, but willing to settle when we needed to. To this day, I mourn the loss of my beloved Dodgers to Los Angeles and will never forgive the Dodgers for deserting me.

I was never a big reader when growing up, but never failed to read the "funnies," the color comic strips in the Sunday newspapers. I don't remember much about what other papers we might have gotten at home, but I do remember the *Sunday Daily News*. I remember that newspaper because on the top of the first page of the funnies pages was my favorite, Dick Tracy. Each week, I devoured the mystery presented in the comic strip. The technology described in the series was sci-fi(ish) like many of the current TV shows which show criminal investigation technology that really doesn't exist. Tracy's critical thinking and use of intellectual curiosity was a model for my career.

I also remember lying on the floor looking up at a console radio and listening to various detective programs. My favorites included "The Shadow," "FBI in Peace and War," and "The Inner Sanctum." I dreamed of being the hero and catching robbers, murderers, and others.

Our home was one of the first to have a television. This magic machine was revolutionary in providing an opportunity to "see" mysteries unfold before our eyes, in my own house! Many of the radio programs morphed onto the small screen. In addition, television presented the opportunity to educate in a way not previously able to reach into the privacy of the home.

In 1954, the first television medical show premiered. Konrad Styner, the physician host of the series played by Richard Boone, became my new hero. He introduced each one of the 51 episodes and appeared in several of them. This award-winning series introduced me to various aspects of medicine that would guide me in my path to a medical career as a poison detective. The show presented both fictional and historically based stories concerning medicine. "Who Search for Truth" was an episode which had a lasting effect on the way I approach a new problem and my attitude about grasping the moment for what it is worth. Styner presented the story of Dr. William Beaumont, an Army physician who found himself caring for Alexis St. Martin, a Canadian trapper who received a gunshot wound to his abdomen, which failed to heal. Beaumont used a non-healing gastro-cutaneous fistula as a "window" into the physiology of digestion. William Beaumont became an historic hero of mine. His ability to seize the moment and by so doing, alter the basic knowledge of human bodily function, became a model for me to emulate.

Another television program I watched regularly, almost religiously, was the police drama *Dragnet*, with its regular unfolding of crimes solved by a pair of Los Angeles police officers. Each week, a new case was revealed in which Sargent Jack Webb and his partner methodically solved each case by interviewing individuals for "just the facts."

There were also a number of other programs that I "had to watch." I was addicted to *Mr. Wizard*. This show, hosted by its creator Don Herbert, was first broadcast in 1951. Herbert played a science hobbyist, and every Saturday morning a neighbor boy or girl would come to visit. The children were played by child actors; oh, how I longed to be one of those visitors. Mr. Wizard always had some kind of laboratory experiment going that taught something about science. The experiments, many of which seemed impossible at first glance, were usually simple enough to be recreated by viewers, and I was always trying to recreate Mr. Wizard's creations, often to the dismay of my family.

I also had a creative streak in my personality and loved to watch the Jon Gnagy show. Gnagy was a self-taught artist whose *Learn to Draw* television show taught millions of Americans how to draw with simple instructions and his "follow me" instruction. I had one of his kits and drew along with him during his regular broadcast programs. There are still times when the creative spark in me breaks out of the clinical shell and allows me to expand my horizons and look for the twists and turns that make medicine truly an art form.

My mother died when I was 11 years old. She came home from shopping one day and laid down for a nap and never woke up. I remember very little about her, only a warm nurturing feeling in my memory bank. I do remember asking her questions, either about things at school or that I wanted to know and her usual answer was "look it up." She didn't just ignore me though, she would ask me how I was doing solving the problem, prodding me along until I solved whatever mystery I had encountered. I also remember asking if I should do one thing or another and her advice was always, I needed to make that decision myself, but should think carefully before deciding. The years after my mother's death consisted of me shuffling back and forth between relatives, and accompanying my father on trips to the

Catskill Mountains, with my sister and my father's single male friends in search of entertainment and female companionship. When I was in junior high school, my father married a teacher in my future high school.

I suppose I seemed to have little or no direction in my life, and my father and new stepmother were concerned that I needed help in choosing a career. The only thing that they saw me really paying attention to was my art and photography, and my father was afraid that I would never earn a living with that, so they sent me to see the high school guidance counselor. I was given the Kuder Preference test. I had to use a stylus to punch out holes in an answer sheet that enabled a counselor to construct a picture encompassing my desires and aptitudes. After I finished the test, I was told that my responses indicated a future as either a police officer or a butler. To say the least I was a bit shaken by this. The counselor explained that I shouldn't take the result literally, that butlers serve people's needs and police officers were problem solvers, so that my direction could certainly be in the area of scientific investigation. Amazing how prescient the test was.

As a junior in high school I chose to be in a special theater arts-related English class. We read plays rather than books. One play that had an enormous effect on my life was Ibsen's *An Enemy of the People*. The lead character in the play, Dr. Stockmann, uncovered the contamination of his town's baths and forced their closure. He was met with resistance from others, including his brother, in his effort to prevent illness by forcing the closure and repairs. In several instances in my career, when I uncovered potentially harmful events, I was met with resistance about the disclosure. To this day, I frequently discuss how one has to stand up for what is right and to protect the innocent people rather than allow yourself to be pushed around by the money influencers.

When planning on college, I really was not given much of a choice. We didn't have a great deal of money and the New York City colleges were essentially tuition-free (a student was responsible for a general fee of $8 per semester and an additional $10 per laboratory course for a lab fee). As I look back on my college decision, I had the opportunity to go to the local college, Brooklyn College from which my sister and stepmother had graduated, travel to the "country" and attend Queens College, or attend an urban school in the form of City College in Manhattan. Alternatively, if I really wanted to be avant-garde, Hunter College, formerly a teachers college and limited to females, had become a liberal arts college and was accepting men. By this time I was willing to state that I wanted to pursue medicine as my career. My father was not 100% supportive of this. His experiences with my mother's death had soured him on the profession, but we didn't fight about it. Tragically, he died during my third year in college, as with my mother, suffering a sudden, catastrophic death. I remember coming home from class and finding him in bed, a little pale and sweaty. I called one of his Masonic brothers, who was an osteopathic physician, somewhat against my father's wishes, and told him what I saw. He was at our house very shortly thereafter. I was in the room when they spoke and the physician examined my father. As he was saying that he didn't find anything to cause him to hospitalize my dad, my father started to grab his chest. I asked if I should leave and the physician said no, he might need me. I remembered that my dad had a small oxygen bottle in his car as he was a dental supply salesman and this was one of the items he carried to demonstrate to his customers. I ran to get it only to return to see my father being unsuccessfully resuscitated. I can still hear the death rattle in my memory today.

As a junior in college I was preparing to apply to medical schools. Although I always seemed to be placed in advanced classes, my grades were never sterling and my GPA not spectacular. I did test well on the Medical College Aptitude Test though, the one thing I really had going for me, besides my passion to pursue a career in medicine. The premedical advisor suggested that I not get my hopes up, because I had too many strikes against me. It was well known that there was religious prejudice and it was difficult for Jewish students, like me, to gain acceptance to medical school. In addition he went on, the fact that I went to a city college and was an "orphan" suggested that there might be insufficient funds available for me to complete school without asking for a scholarship. I managed to graduate from Brooklyn College in 3½ years rather than 4 with well over the minimum credits needed. I attended classes at night and over the summer in order to complete both the required course work for my degree and to apply to medical school as well as take classes that I had an interest in. I took classes in such things as meteorology, television production, and parliamentary procedures. I also worked part-time in the registrar's office helping with such chores as copying transcripts, helping new students register, and at times being a human computer alphabetizing registration cards. I sent applications to both allopathic and osteopathic schools. The physician Masonic friend of my father was an osteopath and he encouraged me to apply to the six osteopathic schools then in existence. I had interviews in both osteopathic and allopathic schools. I remember my very first interview, at the Chicago College of Osteopathic Medicine. It was my very first airplane ride and I was terrified. I managed to get to Chicago a bit shaken but alive. I also had a bit of a problem with the hotel the night before my interview. The bed had what was called 'magic fingers." You put in a quarter and were supposed to get a half hour of massage, really shaking the bed. Unfortunately after 2 hours, the darn bed was still shaking and I couldn't fall asleep, until I found the plug and pulled it out of the electrical socket.

Most interviews consisted of both group interaction activities and individual activities. I remember the interview at the Medical College of Virginia, the school I would eventually attend. They had all of the applicants take the Miller Analogy test. This was a truly amazing experience. I was used to analogy tests from my SAT and MCAT experiences, but this was an analogy test unlike I had ever experienced. I went through the first page and broke out into a cold sweat. Many of the analogies seemed so difficult that I couldn't figure out the answers. After struggling for a while, a pattern emerged for me, they were not simply synonyms or antonyms, etc.; the questions required deconstruction and reconstruction of words, plays on words, and so forth. Once I broke the code, the exam was a breeze, even fun. I found myself laughing out loud, to the consternation of the others who were struggling with the examination with me. Later, on returning to the premedical office and reporting the experience, I was told that Brooklyn College students rarely did well on that test, and they were surprised when they found out that I had done so well. The interview went very well at MCV and they really interested me in taking advantage of the facilities they were developing in such areas as educational television and student involvement in research. I eventually was accepted to three allopathic and one osteopathic schools. I might have been accepted to more had I not withdrawn my applications after deciding that I wanted to go to MCV.

In June, before the start of medical school, I received a letter from MCV describing what matriculating would entail, financially and other. In addition, I received a "reading list." It was suggested that I read the books and articles on the list. I was so overjoyed that I was accepted to the school of my choice, and so frightened that if I didn't read the books I would offend them and would have my acceptance canceled, that I never paused to consider not reading them. I also considered the possibility that there would be a test to see if we read them. I read almost the entire list. Among the books on the list were such classics as *Arrowsmith*, *The Citadel*, *The Green Jungle*, and the book that was to become my "how to succeed in business without even trying" a guide or handbook to my medical career, Berton Roueché's compilation of essays bound together in the book *Eleven Blue Men*.

Roueché wrote articles for the *New Yorker*. In 1944, he was hired as a writer for the magazine. In 1946, "The Annals of Medicine" series in the magazine was created for him. "The Annals of Medicine" was a series about medical detection and the fight against disease. Roueché remained a staff writer for the *New Yorker* until his death, a span of about 50 years. "Eleven Blue Men" was the story of 11 destitute men during the depression who ate at a soup kitchen in New York. Sodium nitrite, corning salt, had been substituted for table salt in making their hot cereal, producing an outbreak of methemoglobinemia, a condition in which the blood becomes cyanotic and the victim turns blue. In 1954 the book *Eleven Blue Men* was published as a compilation of many of his classic essays previously published in the *New Yorker*. An expanded version of the book was published in 1980 as *The Medical Detectives*, thought to be the inspiration behind the popular television show *House*. *The Medical Detectives* has been the muse for many public health individuals. It has taught more people about field epidemiology and the problem-solving aspect of disease investigation than any brick-and-mortar school.

My career has been a romp in the world of Medical Detectives. I have a copy of the book in my office in which I annotate cases that I have dealt with which match Roueché's cases. When asked to organize a 6-week course for medical students in preventive medicine, there was never a hesitation in my mind as to the textbook to use; *The Medical Detectives* was selected. Amazingly, almost every person I know who has been or is involved with epidemiology, preventive medicine, or community health can recite at least chapter names of this book. It is still used in course work around the country by those pursuing degrees and hence careers in public health. I will venture a guess that if you look in the library of every health department and in the possession of every public health field worker, you will find a copy of the book.

As my career matured, and as I amassed my own library of unusual diseases, specifically poisons, I have been asked to give lectures about my experiences. I have been asked so often, "Why don't you write a book?" that the thought crossed my mind that I could emulate the great work of Roueché and help teach the art of diagnosis to individuals in their developing years. In medical school we were always taught that when you hear hoof beats, think horses. My philosophy has always been, yes, do think horses, but remember there might be a time when the horse is a zebra. We also attempt to teach students and residents that if they don't think zebras, they will never know when one goes by them. In certain circumstances, failure to see the first zebra can lead to a stampede that can make many sick, or even die.

It is primarily my love of Roueché's book, married to my personal experiences, that led to my writing these essays. I hope that the readers of this compilation are engaged, and even inspired, the way I was when I first read *The Medical Detectives*. If so, I have succeeded in my endeavors and the legacy of Roueché lives on.

Newark, NJ, USA   Steven M. Marcus

About This Book

The stories I relate in this book are real; they are all cases from my files at the New Jersey Poison Information and Education System. Each chapter is a story about uncovering an unusual toxicological problem. I attempted to recreate these accounts for the reader in the way the cases actually unfolded. The dialogue found in the stories was either transcribed from recordings (as documented in the notes) or was recreated by me, to the best of my memory. The stories are arranged in approximate chronological order. When the individual involved agreed to the use of his or her name, I used their actual name. Of interest, no one refused, but there were many whom I could not reach for their consent. In such cases, I used a fictional name. This book is meant to be read for "fun." I hope it will make learning fun.

Acknowledgments

Antidotes are anti-don'ts unless approved by a qualified healer.

—J. K. Rowling, *Harry Potter and the Order of the Phoenix*

In looking back on my career, there are so many people that I have to thank that it would take another chapter to mention them all. I first credit my parents, whose early deaths cheated them of the knowledge of what I became and the thrill of playing with their grandchildren. They knew just how to push my intellectual curiosity. To my sister, Joelna Marcus, and my stepmother, Rae Marcus, I owe a huge debt for their presence and support through the traumas of the loss of my father and the challenges of my education. My stepmother Rae also was responsible for my starting to date my future wife. She met my future wife's mother at a United Federation of Teachers strike vote and both discussed their children; the rest is history.

Thanks go to the public school system of the City of New York from kindergarten through college, which afforded me a first-class education, all free. To the Medical College of Virginia, whose admissions committee saw something in me that produced my acceptance to their medical school. I also have to mention two specific people from that time of my life. Ralph Tanz still hired me during my "free" semester after finishing college in three and a half years-- knowing that I would probably leave him after only 9 months. Ralph was a professor in the department of pharmacology at New York Medical School at the time and introduced me to experimental pharmacology-- giving me skills that I still depend upon. Interestingly, during my first year in medical school, Ralph moved from academia to the pharmaceutical industry, accepting a position at Geigy Pharmaceuticals, now merged into what is currently known as Novartis. He invited me to spend the summer between my first and second years of medical school with him in his laboratory. Interestingly, there was another student working there, Lewis Goldfrank. Lewis and I drifted apart; he developed his career in Emergency Medicine and Medical Toxicology while I developed my career in Pediatrics and Medical Toxicology. We "found" each other about 20 years later and have been close colleagues in toxicology ever since. Joseph Borzelleca, my pharmacology professor during my second year at the Medical College of Virginia, became my mentor and co-investigator during my medical school career.

My first break in clinical medicine, post my two years in the United States Navy, occurred as the result of meeting a former residency friend from Jacoby Hospital and Albert Einstein College of Medicine, Illana Zarafu, at a meeting of the Society for Pediatric Research. Dr. Zarafu was working as a neonatologist in Newark Beth Israel Medical Center and introduced me to her director, Jules Titelbaum, who hired me as the director of the pediatric clinic and allowed me the flexibility to develop in my areas of interest. My 31 years at The Beth were amazing ones in many ways. Without the continued support and encouragement of Jules and Illana, and the flexibility I had, it is doubtful that my career would have developed the way it did. Sadly, Dr. Zarafu died at too young an age and the department never really seemed the same after that.

I owe a great deal to my college best friend and best man at my wedding, Ronald Ebert, and his wife, Susan, who, living in Boston, were the hidden reason to attend a conference sponsored by the United States Department of Health and Human Services, in Boston, about developing regional poison centers. The program was developed and delivered by Sylvia Micik, a former attending of mine, while I was a resident at Bellevue Hospital. After the conference, I met with Frederick Lovejoy, a faculty member at Harvard University's Medical School. He agreed to take me on as a fellow in medical toxicology at Boston Children's Medical Center and helped to cement my life in toxicology. My thanks to you, Fred and to my co-fellow at the time, and dear friend to this day, Suman Wason and all of the support staff at the Massachusetts Poison Information Center.

My thanks to my colleague and jogging partner during national meetings, William Robertson, the Medical Director of the Washington State Poison Center. He kept pushing me to get more involved and to go for my certification in medical toxicology. Robbie, as he liked to be called, was an amazing positive influence not just on me, but on the entire discipline of medical toxicology. It was an extreme honor to be presented the Ellenhorn Award for achievement in medical toxicology, from the American College of Medical Toxicology, presented to me by Robbie a few years before his death. Thanks to my friend and colleague Barry Rumack, formerly the medical director of the Denver Poison Center and currently on the faculty of the University of Colorado Medical School in Denver, who has always been there for me when I needed answers to questions that puzzle me.

My family was always the most important. To my three children, Jayme, Joshua, and Leigh, I apologize for the missed sporting and school events. I tried to be there for you, but I was often called away to be at a patient's bedside or called to the Department of Health. Where would I be without the most incredible, most important person in my life, my wife and best friend, Amy. I call her a "saint," because putting up with me and my work habits, takes a saintly person. She was instrumental in virtually every career decision I made. She and I are truly partners in life. She has always been my rock, my stability. She suffered through reading every version of every chapter of this book, helping me ensure that the lay person would enjoy reading it as well as the medical professional. She says that she will never eat a piece of fish or meat without thinking about what happened to my patients. In brief, she correctly says that she is the best thing that ever happened to me.

Contents

Introduction

In the mid-1950s, pediatricians in Chicago identified a problem in their community. Children were "accidentally" being exposed to substances in their homes. When the parents either called their physicians or brought the exposed child to an emergency room, there was no easy way to determine what the ingredients were nor what to do about the exposure. A group of pediatricians and pediatricians-in-training went shopping for commercially available products and developed an inventory of ingredients as listed by the manufacturer on the labels. This first poison center then "advertised" its availability to the physicians in the community. This model was replicated by several other communities, and in 1958, the American Association of Poison Control Centers (AAPCC) was established in an effort to build cooperation between these isolated centers. The need for these information services resulted in the expansion of the number of poison centers to a peak of 661 in 1978. By that time, the centers expanded their reach to the lay public as well as to health professionals.

The National Emergency Medical Services Program of 1973 called for the development of a system approach to provide improvement to emergency services and produce a decrease in morbidity and mortality. The goal was to establish regional planning in 15 key areas. Among the components thought to be in need of emergency care under this program were trauma, burns, central nervous system injury, acute cardiac, maternal or infant high risk, acute behavioral (psychiatric) problems, and poisoning.

The New Jersey Department of Health (NJDoH) established a task force to look at the provision of emergency medical services for the state. Enabling legislation was passed in 1982, calling upon the NJDoH to develop a regional drug and poison information system. The New Jersey Poison Information and Education System, a single center, was created from the merging of 32 hospital-based centers and became functional on February 1, 1983. In 2001, the United States Congress passed legislation to stabilize and enhance poison center operations. Through the efforts of the AAPCC, with funding from Congress, a uniform toll-free telephone number (1-800--222-1222) was established as a single point of entry into the poison center system. A call to that telephone number is routed, by geographical location of the caller, to one of fifty-five regional poison centers. Calls are answered by individuals called poison information specialists. They are all nurses, pharmacists, or physicians who are specially trained to deal with telephone calls relating to possible exposures to toxic substances and/or prevention of such. Each center is required to have a medical toxicologist, a physician trained in the discipline of medical toxicology, functioning as the medical director. All calls are documented into an electronic medical record, and abstracts of the calls are uploaded regularly to a national database which has surveillance built in to pick up any potential new toxic emergencies.

The cases discussed in the chapters that follow were all cases called into the New Jersey Poison Information and Education System.

Chapter 1
Forty Blue Kids

The air was crisp and clear, the first cold day of the fall. Wilma Pomerantz awakened with a start as her alarm clock announced the beginning of a new day in the life of a Poison Information Specialist.

A Poison Information Specialist is a nurse, pharmacist, or physician specially trained to answer telephone calls regarding information related to possible poison exposures. This day began like many other days for Wilma: quick clean-up, breakfast, and then the drive to the Information Center, a bank of telephones and computer databases developed to help the specialists respond to a variety of questions from the lay public as well as health professionals throughout the state.

The majority of these calls are related to children who sample their environment by tasting, licking, touching, and, rarely, getting into trouble. As Wilma prepared to go to work, she reflected on previous days of work, wondering what kind of questions would be asked of her today. She finished her breakfast and took a quick look around her house, for she knew it would be thirteen to fourteen hours until she saw it again and wanted to be sure that when she came home after her twelve-and-a-half-hour tour at the Poison Center, there would be nothing for her to do except to prepare for bed, since the work hours are physically as well as intellectually exhausting. The role of the Poison Information Specialist in responding to other people's problems, many of which are perceived by the caller as extremely serious, takes its toll.

The trip to work that day was uneventful as were the first several hours on the job. She responded to run-of-the-mill exposures to silica gel—the little pack of drying agent packaged in such things as shoes—and exposures to various household products and plants in the home. Just before lunch, however, a telephone call came in that would change her day entirely. It was one of those calls that is challenging as well as taxing and requires all of your mental capacity. On the other end of the telephone was a nurse at a Catholic school in New Jersey.

After lunch, and outside for recess, a couple of children entered her office complaining of nausea and headache. Their lips were blue.

"Blue?" asked Pomerantz. "Yes, blue!" replied the nurse.

© Springer International Publishing AG 2017
S.M. Marcus, *Medical Toxicology: Antidotes and Anecdotes*,
DOI 10.1007/978-3-319-51029-3_1

As this was the first cold day of the year, several thoughts flashed through Wilma's mind. Was it cold enough to turn lips blue? Did the children go outside to play without proper clothing on and were their lips blue from circulation decrease because of the cold air? Were there any blueberries in the playground that the children were eating? Was there something blue in the food they ate for lunch?

"No, No, No." The nurse explained that although it was chilly out, it was not cold enough for her to think that the children's lips would be blue from that. Their hands were blue, not just their lips, and the blue coloration would not wipe or wash off. As she spoke to Wilma, one or two children became five or six, then nine or ten, and several of them started vomiting. It became clear that something was seriously wrong. The nurse's office was now in chaos with crying and vomiting children, the ambient noise level rising as the seconds ticked off.

"Contact the parents and let's get them to an emergency room," Pomerantz directed the nurse.

The children began arriving at hospital emergency rooms. At one such hospital, Julia LaJoie, M.D., a pediatric emergency department attending, was the first physician to examine several of the children. The blue discoloration suggested low oxygen levels, which would explain the blue skin color. Julia thought about the basic science of the balance of oxygen in the body.

Oxygen is carried in the blood, reversibly attached to hemoglobin, in the red blood cell and dissolved in the plasma. Red blood cells contain hemoglobin, which contains a porphyrin portion which is a quaternary structure with an iron atom within it. This quaternary structure allows each molecule of hemoglobin to carry four oxygen molecules. The iron atom can exist in two chemical valences, or electrical charge, depending upon the balance of its electrons. In the ferrous, or reduced form, Fe^{2+}, it can "share" an electron with an atom of oxygen (the oxygen acts as an electron donor) and form an "oxygenated" form of hemoglobin, or oxyhemoglobin, giving blood its characteristic red color. Hemoglobin "picks up" this oxygen as blood perfuses the alveolar capillary bed in the lungs and the oxygen breathed in with each breath diffuses across the alveolar plasma membrane. Oxygen obeys the laws of diffusion in that it moves from a high pressure/concentration in the alveolus through the alveolar membrane into the plasma. If the alveolar membrane functions as a perfect permeable membrane, at equilibrium, the oxygen concentration on one side, that is, within the alveolus, should equal that within the plasma. The concentration of oxygen is measured in two terms: in concentration, which relates to the percentage saturation of hemoglobin; and PO_2 which is the partial pressure of oxygen dissolved in the plasma. At normal sea level that is a PO_2 of 100 mmHg and oxygen saturation should reach 100% saturation of hemoglobin in the lungs. This process requires a perfect balance of perfusion, blood supply to and from the alveolar bed, and diffusion of oxygen across the alveolar membrane to maintain the normal state of the organism. The circulatory system then distributes the oxygenated blood to the tissues at which time the oxygen is "dumped," utilized by the tissues in metabolism. With the release of the oxygen, the iron in the hemoglobin is returned to its ferrous state. In the venous side, the oxygen saturation drops to the 40% range, and the blood develops its characteristic blue color in the venous side. The "dumped" oxygen is utilized by the tissues in various metabolic processes. In some disease states, the tissues extract even greater amounts of oxygen from the blood and the oxygen saturation may drop even below that 40%, reflecting the exquisite use of oxygen by the tissues. The blood then gets pumped back to the heart and returns to the lungs to become re-oxygenated.

Some oxygen is, literally, dissolved in the plasma. This constitutes only a very small part of the oxygen used by the tissues of the body. There is a balance between the dissolved oxygen and that bound to hemoglobin in the red cells. Oxygen dissolved in the plasma is said to exert a "partial pressure," which allows oxygen to move across the plasma membrane of the red blood cell and become bound to the hemoglobin within the cell. At a partial pressure of oxygen of 100 mmHg, hemoglobin is 100% saturated and appears to the eye as red. This happens in the lungs, where the PO_2 is 100 mmHg (at sea level). As oxygen is released, "dumped," into the tissues from the plasma, the partial pressure of oxygen drops. This impacts upon the amount of oxygen that hemoglobin can carry. Subsequent to the "loss" of oxygen to the tissues, on the venous side of the circulation, the PO_2 drops to 45 mmHg, and at that partial pressure, hemoglobin is only 40% saturated. Any disease process which interferes with the diffusion of oxygen across the alveolar membrane and into the plasma and then hemoglobin while maintaining the perfusion of that area will interfere with oxygenation and the blood, leaving the lung insufficiently oxygenated.

The relationship between PO_2 and oxygen saturation is plotted on the 'oxygen-hemoglobin dissociation curve,' with PO_2 plotted on the horizontal axis and oxygen saturation (defined as the proportion of maximum amount of oxygen the hemoglobin can carry, with a maximum of 100%) on the vertical access (Fig. 1.1). When one does this, one becomes aware of the non-linearity of the relationship; an "s-shaped curve" is plotted, the oxygen dissociation curve. This is a very important curve, since it displays graphically how hemoglobin acquires and releases oxygen to the fluid and tissues surrounding it.

The drop from a saturation of 100% to that of 60% represents the oxygen that was released into the tissues and made available to tissue cells for metabolism, etc. There is a steep, precipitous drop in saturation when the pressure of oxygen drops below about 60 mmHg, and that is extremely important to remember in protecting a patient from a rapid deterioration in clinical status. A PO_2 of 60 or more can be tolerated by an individual, but any drop below that tends to compromise the patient's clinical status from lack of available oxygen (hypoxemia). There are various influences on the general shape of the oxygen dissociation curve. A "shift to the left" (the top-most curve in Fig. 1.1) denotes an increase in affinity, aka increased binding, of oxygen to hemoglobin and this alteration results in hemoglobin dumping less oxygen at a given PO_2. Note that normally the difference between the oxygen saturation at a PO_2 of 100 and a PO_2 of 40 represents a drop of hemoglobin saturation from 99 to 60%. A shift to the right, as in the bottom-most curve in the figure, denotes less of an affinity and increased dumping of oxygen at a given PO_2, thus a drop from 99.99% saturation at PO_2 of 100 to 55% at a PO_2 of 40, almost 10% more oxygen is available to the tissues. This change in the curve provides a homeostatic mechanism

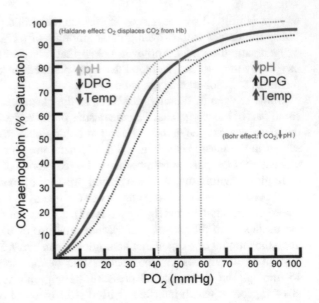

Fig. 1.1 Oxyhaemoglobin dissociation curve. Adapted from an illustration created by Ratznium

to cope with an organism's needs under certain circumstances. For example, when one exercises and the tissues need more oxygen for metabolism, the tissues become more acidic and the body temperature rises. Both are influences that tend to shift the curve to the right causing a decrease in oxygen affinity and increased dumping of oxygen for the tissues. The mnemonic "CADET face Right," has been used by students to help remember this relationship, where C is for CO_2, A for acid, D for 2,3-DPG, E for Exercise, and T for Temperature. Reverse factors, in turn, shift the curve to the left. Among the factors which shift the curve to the left are increasing the affinity for oxygen and decreasing its dumping, include the presence of alkalosis, exposure to carbon monoxide, or, as will soon be seen, the alteration of hemoglobin to methemoglobinemia.

For a patient to develop "cyanosis," a blue discoloration there must be the existence of significant de-oxygenation of the blood. Cyanosis requires the presence of de-oxygenated hemoglobin of more than five grams (hemoglobin is generally measured in grams per 100 mL of blood, a normal individual will have approximately 15 g of hemoglobin, thus to be cyanotic about one third of his/her blood must be in the deoxygenated, or venous-like form), this usually means that the oxygen saturation has dropped below 80%. Such a physical finding leads one to develop a differential diagnosis. Julia rapidly went through this process. If the patient has fluid in his or her lungs, as would happen with an infection such as pneumonia, oxygen will not cross the alveolar membrane as well as it should, since fluid within the alveolar space causes a decrease in the diffusability of oxygen, less oxygen can reach the blood. Having the patient breathe a higher percentage of oxygen will increase the PO_2 in the alveolar space enhancing the diffusion across the alveolar membrane and allow more oxygen to dissolve in the plasma with a consequent increase in hemoglobin saturation and clearing of the cyanosis. She thought about this, and when the children did not "pink up" after being given supplemental oxygen, she pondered where to look next. If blood is shifted from the venous side to the arterial side, a so-called right to left shunt, as occurs in certain congenital heart diseases, the patient will look cyanotic. To see that number of children suddenly developing a right to left shunt would defy the odds of probability.

To check the blood oxygen content of the children in her emergency room, she placed a pulse oximeter probe on the children. A pulse oximeter is a device that measures, non-invasively (not requiring any blood drawing) and indirectly, the oxygen saturation in blood. A sensor is placed on the body, usually on a fingertip or toe, and light of two wavelengths, one usually red, the other infra-red, is passed through the patient's skin to a sensor on the other side of the finger or toe. The absorption of light at these wavelengths differ significantly between arterial (oxygenated) and venous (deoxygenated) blood. The sensor then calculates the ratio of red light measurement to infra-red and calculates the ratio of oxygenated to deoxygenated hemoglobin and the built-in processor converts this ratio to hemoglobin saturation. As stated before, cyanosis usually does not occur until saturation drops below 80%. Julia's suspicions that the children were not absorbing oxygen correctly appeared to be wrong. Although the children were blue, the pulse oximeter showed 88%, a level at which cyanosis, the blue color, is not expected. To explain the degree of blueness of these children, the pulse oximeter should have read below 80%.

Luckily, LaJoie, a recent graduate of the pediatric residency program at Morristown Memorial Hospital, an affiliate of the University of Medicine and Dentistry (now the School of Biomedical and Health Sciences of Rutgers University), had done a rotation at the NJ Poison Control Center and studied "methemoglobinemia," a condition in which blood looks blue in spite of having an oxygen content which should not make the blood blue. She knew that the pulse oximeter reading in cases of methemoglobinemia reads 88%, the same as LaJoie found with these children. She drew blood from the children's arteries and sent the samples to the laboratory for "blood gas evaluation," for confirmation of the methemoglobinemia. The blood gas laboratory has a special piece of equipment, a co-oximeter, which is capable of measuring methemoglobin itself. Having sent the blood to the laboratory she then waited, and waited, and waited for the results. She knew that time was not on her side, and that if she was correct in her thinking, these children needed therapy for their condition, and as quickly as possible. Ten or fifteen minutes later, when she still had not received results, she called the laboratory to find out why. The first technologist she spoke to could not give her an answer to either the level or why the delay. Eventually, the laboratory supervisor told her that she was reluctant to give her the results. She stated that their machine had just been repaired and the technologist felt uncomfortable with the results. Because of the reluctance to trust the results, the lab refused to release the information to her until it was corroborated in another hospital in another laboratory. This was frustrating to LaJoie, so she called me at the poison center.

As circumstances happened, I was in a community clinic at the time, helping children who needed routine care and immunizations in a community-based, safety-net clinic. Pomerantz was able to create a three-way telephone conference between LaJoie, herself, and me.

"Steve, didn't you tell me that a cyanotic individual whose O_2 saturation is normal is suffering from methemoglobinemia until proven otherwise?"

"Yes, I don't remember the conversation but yes, that is true."

"Then why won't the laboratory give me the results?" I had no clue, just a hunch. "Perhaps the results were so high the lab could not believe their own results?"

"Push them, demand the results even if they don't trust them. Call me back with the results and we can discuss them."

By that time several children were being seen in three other hospitals. According to information from the hospitals, when they all in turn called the poison center, all of the children had the same complaints and findings. All were sick with headaches and some with vomiting, but all were various shades of blue with pulse oximeter readings of 88%. Were we being invaded by some weird Smurf disease? Unlikely. The belief by that time was that there was something in the children's environment, most likely something in the environment in the school or in their diet that had caused the outbreak. With the exception of the children treated by LaJoie, the children treated at other hospitals were diagnosed as suffering from "carbon monoxide poisoning" and were treated for that. Although the treatment they were administering, high flow oxygen, would not hurt the children, it would delay the appropriate therapy if they were suffering from methemoglobinemia as LaJoie and I believed. Carbon monoxide poisoning was the diagnosis made at the other hospital emergency room to be the cause because the school's heating system had just been turned on for the first time that day. The physicians were attributing the children's illness to exposure to this gas. The treating hospitals believed that carbon monoxide had leaked from the school's heating system.

As the Poison Center became involved with the three hospitals, the center attempted to explain to the hospitals that it is unusual for a patient suffering from carbon monoxide poisoning to be blue. Carboxyhemoglobin, the form of hemoglobin in which carbon monoxide (rather than oxygen) is attached to hemoglobin, maintains the usual reddish tint and shifts the oxy-hemoglobin dissociation curve to the left, decreasing the release of bound oxygen from hemoglobin. Many textbooks describe a "cherry-red" appearance (which is more appropriate when describing a victim who dies from carbon monoxide poisoning rather than a live victim, because the oxygen stays bound to hemoglobin after death and thus maintains the red appearance to the victim's blood and tissues rather than the usual blue discoloration found at death because of lack of circulation). We explained that we believed the children were suffering from methemoglobinemia, not carbon monoxide poisoning. Although, at that time, we could not explain why a group of children going out to play after lunch would suddenly develop methemoglobinemia, I felt that this was the working diagnosis.

By mid-afternoon, there were forty children in three hospitals. The majority of them were at the hospital closest to the school, some at a more distant hospital, and the remainder at Julia's hospital. By 5:00 p.m., the laboratory confirmed the diagnosis of methemoglobinemia, with levels ranging from 15 to 40% (normal is less than 3% and over 25% potentially life-threatening).

Methemoglobin is an abnormal type of hemoglobin, the oxygen-carrying component of red blood cells. It can exist as either a congenital (inborn and inherited) or acquired form. Congenital forms of methemoglobin consists of two types, one an abnormality in the formation of the basic hemoglobin molecule itself, in which the amino acid tyrosine replaces histidine, which then binds to globin. This aberrant combination permits oxidation of the iron within the molecule, resulting in an abnormal hemoglobin called congenital "hemoglobin M." The other form of congenital methemoglobinemia consists of a defect in the enzyme which maintains a normal level of methemoglobin produced by normal metabolism within the body. The normal concentration of methemoglobin is 1–3% and is not associated with any clinical symptoms. The enzyme diaphorase (also known as NADH-methemoglobin reductase, also known as cytochrome b5 reductase) working with the co-enzyme nicotinamide adenine dinucleotide (NAD) in its reduced version, NADH, which is produced by normal aerobic metabolism in the body [NAD + H$^+$ + 2 electrons yields NADH], reduces the "normally" produced methemoglobin and keeps the concentration "normal" (see Fig. 1.2). Deficiency of this enzyme can occur through inheritance. Methemoglobin reductase deficiency exists in two forms, a less severe form which exists only in the red blood cells and a second which exists in all cells in the body. The former is associated with persistent methemoglobinemia but appears not to affect longevity while the latter is associated with numerous other abnormalities and compromised life expectancy. It would be unlikely that 40+ children would suddenly present with congenital deficiencies.

NADH-Methemoglobin reductase can become "overwhelmed" when some oxidative "stress" causes the iron in the hemoglobin molecule, normally in the ferrous state, or 2+ charge, to lose an electron and become oxidized into the ferric state, 3+ charge, methemoglobin. The list of such stress factors is extremely long, including various chemicals and drugs. Methemoglobin is unable to carry oxygen to the extent that normal, unoxidized hemoglobin does. Pulse oximeters, the device used to measure oxygen saturation in the first case, are widely used devices which depend upon calculating the ratio between hemoglobin with and without oxygen by shining a

Fig. 1.2 Stress-induced oxidation of hemoglobin into methemoglobinemia and the homeostatic reduction of methemoglobin to hemoglobin by methemoglobin reductase, which requires the presence of NADH

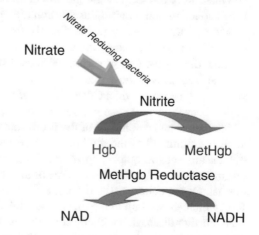

special light-emitting diode on the skin. The skin color is then "read" at different wave lengths, slightly different shades of red. Methemoglobin disturbs the normal ratio and produces a "false" result. The laboratory analyzes oxygen in a slightly different way. The machine used is called a blood gas analyzer and measures oxygen dissolved in the fluid compartment of the blood with a special oxygen probe and also measures methemoglobin with a co-oximeter, similar to the way the pulse oximeter is used in the emergency room. The measurement of dissolved oxygen as is measured in the laboratory is reported as the partial pressure of oxygen in the blood (PO_2). Since methemoglobin only disturbs oxygen carried by the hemoglobin in the red cell and not in the plasma, dissolved oxygen is unaffected, thus the PO_2 may be normal or close to it. In non-methemoglobin states one would not expect to see cyanosis in a patient unless the PO_2 is below 60 mm, 3/5 of the normal.

When the laboratory finally reported the results, the PO_2 was in fact over 100 mmHg, much too high to account for the blue discoloration of the children. Not only does methemoglobin not carry as much oxygen as regular hemoglobin, but the ability to dump oxygen from the blood into the tissues is reduced by the interference with this process, resulting in a change in the shape of the oxygen dissociation curve. This situation produces a combination problem which produces clinical symptoms which can result in death if not treated correctly and promptly.

Wilma and I spoke to the treating physicians at the hospitals to help them with the appropriate management of methemoglobinemia. I became so concerned about the extent of the outbreak, and what I believed to be the misdirected therapy, that I finished up the in the clinic, hopped into my car—my "blue bomber," as we affectionately called it—and sped off to the hospitals. I was told that several of the staff from the school were with the children at one of the hospitals, so rather than go to where LaJoie was, I elected to go there, in hope that I could establish an etiological basis for the outbreak.

Speaking to the school staff, my goal was to determine what, if anything, the children had been exposed to which stressed their hemoglobin and turned them blue. The playground was not down-wind from any particular commercial facility and there were no methemoglobinemia inducing plants or substances in the vicinity. I then concentrated on what the children did prior to recess.

Most of them went to recess directly from their lunch. There were two lunch periods, so I needed to determine if there was any difference between the children who ate during the first or second periods. I developed a table listing the children who became ill and those that did not into first and second lunch periods. To my surprise, it became evident that only children who ate during the second lunch period became sick. I then did some further problem solving. I developed a table which had in one column all of the foods that the children who got sick ate, and in another column all of the food that children who did not get sick ate. As it turned out, the answer was quickly apparent, all the children who were sick had eaten soup during the second lunch period. Some of the children who ate soup, however, stayed normal. Of the children who did not eat soup, none became ill. There was no other food which showed up in the diets of all the sick children and not in the well children. Further discussion with the children and their parents determined that only the children who had second helpings of the soup became sick.

The soup was a commercially produced and purchased chicken noodle soup, from a major manufacturer. I requested that leftover soup be bottled and saved. I also requested that the empty containers from the implicated soup be retained, and that their code numbers be compared with unopened cans so that we could compare analyses of both used and unused soup containers. As luck had it, the code numbers of involved soup and unopened containers matched.

"I would never add anything to the children's soup. I wouldn't want to risk the health of any of the children," was the response of the sister who functioned as the Catholic school's cook. I grew up in Brooklyn, a "nice Jewish boy" in a mixed religion neighborhood. Many of my childhood friends attended Catholic parochial schools. My friends told me many stories about their interactions with the nuns at their school and taught me never to cross a nun. So I was not about to pressure the "chef." The cook told me that the soup was served directly out of the can and that nothing had been added to it. I remembered reading an article, "Eleven Blue Men," a classic medical detective story by Berton Roueché, about eleven homeless men served porridge which had accidentally been "salted" with saltpeter (sodium nitrite) rather than salt (sodium chloride). These men turned blue, just like our children. I was concerned that since so many people put extra salt in chicken noodle soup, perhaps this had happened here. I asked again, "Was any salt added to the soup or made available to the children?" Again the cook replied, "I told you I would never do anything to hurt the children."

To treat their methemoglobinemia, methylene blue, a blue dye, was administered to the children. This substance, working with a proton, hydrogen, from the reduced form of Nicotinamide adenine dinucleotide phosphate (NADPH) produced by the "hexose monophosphate shunt," reduces methemoglobin producing an oxidized methylene blue, leukomethylene blue, converting the methemoglobin back to regular hemoglobin (see Fig. 1.3). Administering a blue dye to a blue patient and seeing the patient turn pink, is an amazing experience. Seeing it over and over again in a cluster of children in an emergency room is something one never forgets. That is exactly what happened to the children involved in this outbreak: we turned our forty little blue children pink by giving them doses of a blue dye. The methylene blue was then eliminated from the blue children's bodies through their kidneys, in their urine, turning it blue-green, to the amazement of everyone involved. Had the methylene blue not worked—that is, had the children not reverted from their blue coloration to pink—we would have considered either an error in diagnosis, unlikely given the eventual readings of methemoglobin levels as high as forty-five, or the possibility of glucose-6-phosphate dehydrogenase deficiency, also known as G6PD deficiency. This inherited condition exists in two forms: a severe form in which the enzyme is absent or very nearly so and usually presents with acute hemolysis of red blood cells (destruction in the circulation), or a less severe form in which there is only partial deficiency and the hemolysis is usually not severe. About 10% of the African American population has the milder form of G6PD deficiency. This enzyme is required in the first step of the hexose monophosphate shunt, thus lack of the enzyme results in lower concentrations of the NADPH required to convert methylene blue to leukomethylene blue, which is then responsible for the reduction of methemoglobin. If there is no response to treatment because of this deficiency, then the only

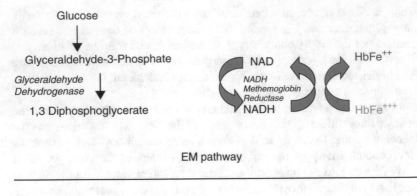

EM pathway

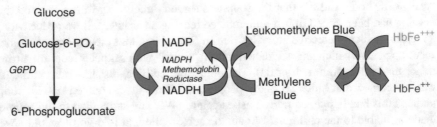

Hexose monophosphate shunt

Fig. 1.3 Comparison of the reduction of methemoglobin to hemoglobin. The usual homeostatic mechanism is with NADH requiring methemoglobin reductase. The mechanism involved with the use of the antidote, methylene blue, requires NADPH

treatment available is an exchange transfusion, a tedious and potentially dangerous procedure in which the blood of the victim is removed and exchanged for other blood which does not have methemoglobin. Such blood is exchanged in aliquots, or fractions, usually 25–50 mL a time. It is important that young blood be used, since the concentration of the enzyme, G6PD, decreases substantially over time.

After further discussion with the involved students and faculty, it was determined that there was no other food that could be related to the outbreak of the disorder. By this time, the State Department of Health was involved, as was the Division of Consumer Products. It was feared that the original soup in the containers might be contaminated with a chemical, specifically saltpeter or sodium nitrite, commonly used to "cure" beef. This substance has been confused historically with salt and produced outbreaks of methemoglobinemia. The Department of Health embargoed the open soup, unfinished quantities of the prepared soup, and the unopened containers.

I was convinced that the source of the outbreak was the soup. Believing the cook, I feared that the soup was contaminated in production and asked the state to analyze the soup immediately. I was told that it would be done the first thing in the morning. I found this to be totally unacceptable. I needed to know immediately what caused the outbreak and if it was the soup. We needed to determine if the unopened cans were contaminated. If so we were faced with a possible nationwide public health emergency and we would have to do something to warn the public. I tried my best to convince the public health officials, to no avail. Years earlier I had developed a collegial friendship with a senior physician at the New Jersey Department of Health, Leah Ziskin, M.D. Luckily I had her office and home telephone numbers. Frustrated by what I believed to be the intransigence of the public health people I had been dealing with, I called Dr. Ziskin.

"Hi, Leah," I stated, "how are you?"

"Just fine," she replied. "I hear that you are involved in an outbreak involving a group of children."

"Yes, I have over forty children suffering from methemoglobinemia, and I think the soup that they ate was the source of the intoxication, although I have no clue how the soup could have been contaminated. The chef, a nun, says that nothing was added to the soup, that she heated it directly out of the can. I am worried that the soup, made by a New Jersey company, could have been contaminated during manufacture."

"I already spoke to the laboratory people," she said. "They assured me," she stated, "it will be analyzed the first thing in the morning."

"I really want it analyzed immediately. How can we justify waiting until tomorrow?" I replied.

"I understand your involvement in the case and your need for instant gratification," Ziskin responded, "but opening the lab and doing the analysis off hours is just not going to happen."

"You have me wrong, Leah," I responded. "Imagine the possibility that, while we sleep, someone in California or elsewhere develops methemoglobinemia and dies after drinking this soup, and someone finds out that we had decided to wait until the morning to analyze the soup, how would we feel then?"

That night, the state laboratory analyzed the open soup and the unopened soup. The nitrite concentration of the open soup was extremely high while the nitrite concentration of the unopened cans was negligible. Dr. Ziskin called me at home to relate the results to me. To say the least I was relieved at the determination that the intact soup was not the source of the contamination, but this left me to find out how the soup became contaminated. I knew that I would have to confront the nun-chef in the morning. That led to a sleepless night.

The following day, the local Department of Health went to the school and examined the plumbing system, since the water supply of the school came from municipal water. Tap water throughout the school was analyzed and no significant nitrite concentration was found. Records of repairs done in the school were reviewed and it was determined that one week prior to the outbreak the heating system had undergone its annual repair and safety check, and an anti-corrosive agent was added to the boiler. The anti-corrosive agent was a combination of sodium borate and sodium nitrite and, rather than emptying the boiler completely, this anti-corrosive agent was added to the water already in the boiler. When analyzed by the state lab, the soup had high concentrations of borate as well as nitrite. This established an apparent link between the boiler water and the soup.

The school had a steam heating system. Water in the boiler is heated until it gets to "steam" temperature, and then the steam rises in the heating pipes to the radiators throughout the school. The steam pushes the air within the pipes out through valves in the radiators until the heat of the steam closes the valves. In this process, some steam is always lost, producing the characteristic "hiss" heard. After the heat in the radiator raises the ambient temperature to whatever has been set for it, the school's thermostat turns off the boiler, allowing the steam to cool back into water, which then falls back though the pipes into the boiler. Invariably some water is thus lost from the boiler and must periodically be replaced. In private homes there is usually a valve which has to be manually opened to allow water from the municipal water supply and refills the boiler to its critical level. In many large buildings this is done automatically by a procedure which mirrors the manual private home system, but the valve automatically opens and allows fresh water to pour into the boiler when the boiler senses the water level is too low. Normal engineering controls include a "check valve" between the boiler system and the potable water within an institution to avoid excess water going into the boiler and prevent boiler water from escaping into the institution's potable water supply. When inspected, it appeared that the check valve was old and in need of replacement, and at the time of the inspection appeared dysfunctional. In reviewing the circumstances of the event, the likely explanation was that water was added from the kitchen tap to the soup, and at that time the broken check valve was in the "open" position at the exact time that the boiler was firing, creating a pressure differential between the boiler and the kitchen sink leading to movement of water from the boiler (high pressure area) into the kitchen sink (low pressure area). Thus, the soup became contaminated with water from the boiler instead of water from the municipal water supply. Meanwhile, the nun continued to insist that she didn't add anything to the soup—who was I to confront the nun?

A new check valve was installed and the school reopened with no new incidents occurring.

When I presented Sister Anne (pseudonym) with all of this evidence in my hands, she stated, "I only used a little water to '*stretch* the soup.'"

Note: The dialogue in this chapter is recreated from notes in the Poison Center's medical records, on file digitally and on microfiche at the New Jersey Poison Information and Education System.

Suggested Reading

Bradbury S. Methaemoglobinemia. Medicine. 2011;40(2):59–60.

Jain MD, Nikonova A. Methemoglobinemia from curing salt. Can Med Assoc J. 2013;185(16):E771.

Shih RD, Marcus SM, Genese CA, et al. Methemoglobinemia attributable to nitrite contamination of potable water through boiler fluid additives—New Jersey, 1992 and 1996. MMWR. 1997;46(9):202–4.

Chapter 2
Something's Fishy

The telephone rang early one morning at my desk at the New Jersey Poison Information and Education System. As was my habit, I was reviewing the previous day's cases called into the poison center. It was Elvis Perez on the line. Elvis, a certified poison information specialist who was trained as a nurse and had spent the last several years fielding the telephones at the hotline for drug and poison information, had a doctor on the line with some questions that he felt I should handle. Dr. Goldsmith was calling about a 38-year-old woman who had come to his office on October 11 with what he thought were strange, unrelated complaints. She explained to him that her hands felt as if they were burning, and that she felt weak and had a metallic taste in her mouth. Dr. Goldsmith had done routine laboratory work, which did not help him make a diagnosis. When she returned to his office a week later, she was complaining of a continuation of those symptoms but now also had extreme fatigue, itching all over, excess tearing, and pain in her eyes. She was so sensitive to light that she resorted to wearing sunglasses most of the time. She had searched the Internet and asked him to check her for mercury poisoning. He read her laboratory results for me: chemistry profile normal; complete blood count normal; Lyme titer by immunoassay screening test was 1.81, but specific testing by a more precise test was negative; a blood mercury level was abnormal with a result of 29.8 µg/L (normal for environmental exposure is less than 15 and should not be greater than 15 at the end of a shift if there is an occupational exposure). We spoke about the interpretation of her results and the usual symptoms of mercury poisoning. He knew of no obvious exposure that his patient had to mercury. She was a graduate student and no member of her family worked with mercury.

We discussed the controversy regarding mercury in dental fillings and the fact that scientists are somewhat divided on whether there is enough mercury liberated from such fillings to represent any potential hazard. There is some data to suggest that that soon after a filling is placed in a tooth there may be some absorption of mercury but that this appears to decrease rapidly and produces no obvious ill effects. We also discussed the fact that removal of the patient's fillings might represent a greater risk than leaving them intact. Further, we discussed the fact that her mercury

© Springer International Publishing AG 2017
S.M. Marcus, *Medical Toxicology: Antidotes and Anecdotes*,
DOI 10.1007/978-3-319-51029-3_2

level may have been dietary in nature and that she should be placed on a diet free of shellfish and other fish for several days. After such a period with no fish consumption, a collection of all her urine for twenty-four hours should be analyzed for mercury to see if she really had a high mercury level in her body.

Calomel (mercurous chloride) was once a commonly used medication. It was thought to increase the flow of bile and urine and was used as the treatment for syphilis for several hundred years until its toxicity became apparent. Benjamin Franklin was reported by some to have been the source of the phrase "a night with Venus, a lifetime with Mercury." Mercury, as mercuhydrin, was a commonly used diuretic to increase urine flow until forty years ago, when safer alternatives became available. Mercuric chloride was commonly used as a topical antiseptic solution. This preparation was dispensed in unique, dark blue-grey, irregularly shaped "pills" which were, roughly, in the shape of a coffin and were labeled with the word *poison* on one side and a skull and crossbones on the other. Mercury in its organic form, Mercurochrome, was and still is, commonly found in homes and used as an antiseptic on minor wounds. Mercury salts, as dusting powder, are frequently still used as protection against mold, etc. on seeds, particularly wheat and corn. The mistaken use of these for food preparation has led to several outbreaks of mercury poisoning, such as during the 1970s in Iraq. Acute mercury poisoning is extremely unusual today. When it does occur, it is usually the result of a suicide attempt. The symptoms of acute poisoning usually start with severe vomiting and diarrhea, which may include large quantities of blood. Loss of fluid and blood through the diarrhea may be so profound as to produce shock and rapid demise. One of the most famous outbreaks of chronic mercury poisoning occurred from the contamination of Minamata Bay in Japan with methylmercury. Two young girls were seen by physicians in Minamata City. The physicians were puzzled by their symptoms: difficulty walking, difficulty speaking, and . It was initially thought to be an infectious disease, something like polio, which occurred in epidemic proportions throughout the world at the time. Serendipitously, anecdotes of a strange phenomenon in the community began to appear. Something peculiar was happening to the wildlife and specifically to the cat population. Cats, often allowed to eat the leftover fish, developed seizures, were "going mad" and dying. Locals called it the "cat dancing disease." This eventually led to the finding of the contamination of the bay by the industrial release of methylmercury into the bay. The contamination was devastating to the population. By the time the outbreak was uncovered and the release of mercury stopped, over 2300 individuals became afflicted and nearly half succumbed to the effects. Exposure of fetuses in utero led to a severe form of cerebral palsy, the subject of a *Life* magazine photo essay by the famous US photographer Eugene Smith entitled "Death-Flow from a Pipe." Chronic mercury poisoning has often been the result of an occupational exposure. Hatters used mercury to cure leather into felt during the nineteenth century. Those in hat production were exposed to large quantities of liquid mercury over protracted periods of time. Such chronic occupational exposure led to such peculiar symptoms as feeling that teeth are loose in the jaw, slurred speech, memory loss, rapid swings in emotions (a person may be laughing one minute and crying the next), assorted aches and pains, tremors, and a metallic taste in the mouth. The symptom of erratic behavior, embodied by Lewis Carroll's Hatter character in *Alice's Adventures in Wonderland*, has led to the phrase "mad as a hatter." Patients often complain of difficulty paying attention and have a tremor which interferes with their handwriting.

Two weeks later Dr. Goldsmith called me with the twenty-four-hour urine mercury level. This time the mercury studies of the patient, Darlene Hanson, were normal; she excreted only 6 μg of mercury in a full twenty-four hours. It was clear that her diet had been responsible for her prior abnormal tests. We spoke about other possible causes of her symptoms, and I offered to see her in consultation if she felt it necessary. Two hours later the patient called the office and we had a nice discussion about her problems. She had been in good health until vacationing with her family in the Caribbean. The family spent several weeks there during the preceding summer. The family had a grand time enjoying the activities available and became familiar with the local foods. They loved the silver snapper served there so much that they brought some of the fish home with them and froze it. On October 5, she cooked the fish for a family dinner. Her husband did not eat the fish because he thought it was too spicy, but both the patient and her daughter ate a full meal of fish, vegetable, and salad. The following day the fish was used to prepare a fish stew and the entire family ate it. She continued to eat the fish for the following days. On the day after consuming the fish, her daughter developed abdominal cramping, nausea, dizziness, and pains in both of her ankles and groin. The gastrointestinal symptoms disappeared spontaneously but the ankle pains continued off and on. On the fourth day after the fish meal, Darlene developed diarrhea, generalized aches and malaise, sweating, and the feeling of tingling of her tongue and lips. She complained of memory loss and a severe metallic taste in her mouth, which prompted her to ask for the mercury studies. She thought that she had gone a bit crazy, because she stated that soon after she developed these symptoms she noticed that hot coffee or tea seemed cold, and cold felt hot to her. We set up an appointment for the following week. This constellation sparked my interest. I had been involved in several cases just like this. The first case I became involved with occurred in the late 1970s in a physician who developed the identical symptoms after eating red snapper on a trip to the Caribbean. She became ill, while her husband did not. Yet another case involved a television producer who shared a meal of grouper with a priest after completing an educational television show; the producer became ill, the priest showed no signs of illness.

I saw Ms. Hanson on October 31. She came accompanied by her husband and daughter. On the day I saw her, she was complaining of tingling in her tongue and lips, memory loss, photophobia, and itching in her ears as well as pain in her ankles. I made the presumptive diagnosis of ciguatera fish poison.

According to the U.S. Centers for Disease Control, ciguatera is the most frequently reported food poisoning related to the ingestion of fish. It is commonly found contaminating fish that live in warm water and feed at reefs, such as in Hawaii, Florida, the Caribbean, and the Indian and South Pacific oceans. There are over 100 fish species reported to harbor the toxin responsible for the poisoning. The list includes grouper, snapper, dolphin, trigger, barracuda, parrot fish, Spanish mackerel, mullet, kole, and many more. The toxin is produced by a tiny micro-organism known as a dinoflagellate. The small, blue-green protozoan (single-cell organism) *Gambierdiscus toxicus* and bacteria within it are thought to be responsi-ble for the production of the toxin. The production appears to increase during times of algal blooms, such as red or green tides. These dinoflagellates are the food of smaller fish, generally herbivorous (plant-eating) fish. These fish then are the prey of larger carnivorous fish and so on up the food chain until a human ingests the fish. Generally, the larger the fish, the older the fish—and the more likely that it has ingested considerable toxin. In this way the toxin is bio-amplified and can reach toxic levels and cause illness when ingested by an unwary human. There probably are a diversity of toxins, since at least three toxins have already been identified. This helps account for variations in the clinical effects seen. The toxin is not destroyed by heat or freezing, and it is colorless, odorless, and tasteless. It does not disturb the taste of the fish. People have developed symptoms after eating fish boiled, broiled, fried, barbecued, or raw.

The toxin produces neurological and, potentially, cardiac abnormalities, by inter-fering with the way nerve impulses are transmitted. A normal nerve or muscle cell stays in its resting stage through several means of balancing the concentration of certain metallic ions on both sides of the cell membrane. There are a series of tiny pumps and channels which are responsible for maintaining the status quo of the cells in the body, particularly the central nervous system. Virtually every cell in the body contains what is termed the sodium-potassium ATPase pump. Sodium is pumped out of a cell and potassium is pumped in, but slightly unequally, in that more sodium ions are pumped out then potassium ions are pumped in. There is, thus, always an imbalance and a slight electrical charge across the membrane, as in a battery. When an electrical impulse, in the form of a nerve impulse, hits the cell, the pump stops functioning momentarily, resulting in sodium ions rapidly rushing into the cell and potassium ions rushing out. As the impulse passes, the pump then pumps sodium out and potassium in. The cell then returns to its resting state. If the cell is a muscle cell, the rapid movement of sodium into the cell causes the muscle to contract; if a nerve cell, the change in electrical activity allows the impulse to continue along the path of the nerve jumping to another nerve, etc. The ciguatera toxin distorts this delicate balance with the effect that the cell membrane appears to be more permeable to sodium, allowing more sodium to build up inside the cell and causes the cell to be more excitable. In a "slight of evolution," the infected fish is missing the binding site for the toxin, and thus cannot become affected by the toxin while it becomes a depot for the toxin. The toxin accumulates in the muscles of the fish. As the fish ages and eats more toxin-contaminated smaller fish, the concentra-tion of toxin increases. The toxin is colorless, odorless, and tasteless, so the hapless victim has no idea that he or she has become poisoned until the classical symptoms and signs develop.

The history of exposure and development of symptoms is highly variable. The diagnosis is usually made only after the full-blown neurological effects are evi-dent. The meal usually is unremarkable. The first symptoms may be abdominal in nature: cramping, vomiting, and diarrhea. These may occur within two to six hours but may be delayed for twenty-four hours in some circumstances. Headaches, sweating, tearing of the eyes, and pain on looking into lights are common as is numbness of the tongue, lips, and throat. A metallic taste is often reported by those affected. By far the most striking complaint is the peculiar hot–cold reversals so characteristic of this intoxication. Patients often describe pain or burning of their arms or legs. Muscle aches and weakness may occur. Occasionally, muscle weakness may be so severe that a victim is bedridden. Toxin in pregnant women affected by ciguatera may cross the placenta and produce abnormalities in the fetus. Breastfeeding mothers have been reported to contaminate their infants by nursing. There are reports of men complaining of penile discomfort after having vaginal sex with a woman suffering from symptoms of the toxin. The reverse has also been reported—that is, a woman complaining of vaginal pain and discomfort after sex with a man who harbors the toxin.

Treatment of the symptoms is not very effective. If suspected shortly after eating a meal, some toxin may be forced out through the urine. A diuretic is often prescribed to enhance urinary flow. The most often reportedly used is mannitol, a sugar which remains in the blood stream rather than being distributed into the tissues and draws water from the tissues into the plasma volume and increases urine tubular flow. It is unlikely that the toxin can be removed after twenty-four hours. Amitriptyline has been reported, in some cases, to be successful in reversing some of the symptoms. This drug appears to block the channels through which sodium moves, the sodium channel, and thus closes the path that the sodium ions move through. The list of other therapies tried and techniques used to remove toxin is very long, suggesting that no one approach has stood the test of time. This may be secondary to the fact that there is usually a mixture of toxins involved rather than a single one. The symptoms are usually self-limited. Recovery may not be complete for many years. Repeated exposure to the toxin seems to amplify the disability.

I gave Ms. Hanson a prescription for amitriptyline, an anti-depressant medication which has sodium-channel-blocking effects and has been found effective in similar cases. She was given an appointment to return the following week, and I asked her to bring some of the remaining fish with her so that it could be sent out for analysis.

The following week she was still complaining of the tingling of her tongue and joint pains. She continued to have problems concentrating but her appetite had improved. I increased her dose of medication and made a follow-up appointment for the following week.

The next week found her in much better spirits. She had been able to go to the supermarket and picked up a cold soda which felt cold to her. She stated that although she was still forgetful, her mind seemed less foggy.

At the one month follow-up visit, she was complaining of side effects of the drug: blurred vision, dry mouth, problems urinating, and constipation. Over the next months I adjusted her dose depending on her symptoms and the presence of side effects. The hot–cold reversals disappeared as did the joint pains. She continued to have "up and down" days.

Two years later she was able to stop the medication.

The fish sample that she gave to me was sent to the laboratory of Dr. Yoshitsugi Hokama, Professor of Pathology at the University of Hawaii at Manoa. The laboratory reported that two pieces of fish tested positive for ciguatoxin on an immunoassay. The fish was subjected to chemical breakdown so that it could be administered in liquid form and in a controlled concentration to experimental mice and guinea pigs. The extract killed the mice rapidly. On an experimental guinea-pig model in which the heart of the animal was treated with the extract, the heart rate dropped and the force of the contraction of the heart muscle decreased. Both of these effects were prevented by a substance which is thought to have the exact opposite effect of ciguatera.

There is a test available to detect toxin in fish before it is sold to the user. Unfortunately it is not yet widely used. Since the age of the fish is related to the potential for contamination, it may be advisable to limit fish intake to smaller, younger fish. I only chance eating a full fillet rather than part of a fish. Eating fish during a red or green algal bloom may not be wise.

We are told to decrease our intake of beef to prevent coronary heart disease, chicken may give us salmonella poisoning, vegetables and fruit may be contaminated with viral hepatitis, etc. From this experience, it may not be safe to turn to fish. That doesn't leave much choice. I suppose all we can do is be vigilant and hope that if we become sick, there will be a knowledgeable physician to make the diagnosis and intervene to prevent a long-term disability.

Suggested Reading

Dickey R, Plakas S. Ciguetera: a public health perspective. Toxicon. 2010;56:123–36.

Friedman M, Fleming LE, Fernandez M, et al. Ciguetera fish poisoning: treatment, prevention and management. Mar Drugs. 2008;6:456–79.

Graber N, Stavinsky F, Hoffman R, et al. Ciguetera fish poisoning—New York City, 2010–2011. Morb Mortal Wkly Rep. 2013;62(4):61–5.

Pennotti R, Scallan E, Backer L, et al. Ciguetera and scombroid fish poisoning in the United States. Foodborne Pathog Dis. 2013;10(12):1059–66.

Chapter 3
Cold as a Fish on Ice

After the February 1993 bombing of New York's World Trade Center, both law enforcement and the medical community began preparing for further potential terrorist attacks. National programs were developed to prepare healthcare facilities to respond to victims of biological and chemical terrorist activities. Although this particular event occurred a few years before the World Trade Center attack of 2001, it was several years after the Aum Shinrikyo sarin attack in Tokyo. The belief that there might someday be a biological or chemical terrorist attack in the United States led to the development of training programs for emergency responders and healthcare workers in dealing with such terrorist attacks and with substances which might be used. At the time of this incident, training had already been completed for all emergency medical service providers about the potential use of nerve agents as terrorist weapons. First responders and emergency department providers all were required to attend educational programs and to develop protocols to both respond to the victims and to protect themselves and their facilities from the effects of such agents of mass destruction.

In the shadow of these events, the Poison Center received a call from the emergency department of a hospital requesting advice on how to prepare to treat a patient suspected of having ingested a lawn product which was thought to contain both insect and disease control substances. Understanding that many of these products are close relatives of the nerve agents used as weapons of terrorist activities the physicians were seeking advice. The emergency department physician said that he had little information but had been told that a local first aid squad, a so-called basic life support unit, had responded to a call for help and found a patient unresponsive with a pulse of fifty and pupils six mm wide. The squad requested that an advanced life support team respond. A mobile intensive care unit was dispatched. The mobile intensive care team arrived and found the patient on the floor of his garage, unresponsive to commands. The paramedic who examined him said that the patient's lungs "sounded wet" and the patient's pupils were two mm in diameter (very constricted). The assumption was that, given the circumstances as to how he was found and the presence of a lawn product in the garage which contained both an insecticide

© Springer International Publishing AG 2017
S.M. Marcus, *Medical Toxicology: Antidotes and Anecdotes*,
DOI 10.1007/978-3-319-51029-3_3

and a lawn disease preventer, that the victim had ingested this product. The physician was looking for help in preparing his team in advance of the patient's arrival.

Considering the physical findings and the circumstances of the possible exposure, the working diagnosis was an exposure to a pesticide which affects the nervous system, an organophosphate or carbamate chemical. These chemicals have the same effect as the chemical warfare agents known as "nerve gases."

Within all nerve-cell endings are vesicles, like tiny containers in the cell, which contain the chemical acetylcholine, which is called a neuro-transmitter. When a nerve impulse reaches the nerve cell, these vesicles migrate to the inner membrane of the nerve cell at the junction with either another nerve cell or a muscle cell. Once at the inner border, the vesicle attaches and then opens into the space between that nerve cell and the next and releases its acetylcholine into the cleft between the cells, also known as the synaptic cleft. This allows the propagation of the nerve impulse to the next cell by causing a depolarization of that cell. There is a chemical produced by the body which then metabolizes the acetylcholine in the synaptic cleft and thus terminates the impulse. This chemical is termed acetylcholinesterase. I like to think of it as "Pacman" gobbling up the acetylcholine. The "nerve agents," regardless of their use as pesticides or warfare agents, work in the same way, by inactivating acetylcholinesterase. If the acetylcholine stays in the synaptic cleft, the cell cannot recover from the depolarization and doesn't relax. If many of the junctions between nerves and muscles are depolarized the muscle is then paralyzed and incapable of further contraction. The muscle may seem to be continually contracting, it may actually take on the look of a bag of worms moving around, a reaction called fasciculation.

Many garden insecticides contain chemicals which possess the ability to inactivate acetylcholinesterase. The clinical picture of a poisoning from such an agent reveals the overstimulation of the nervous system which uses acetylcholine as its neurotransmitter, known as the autonomic nervous system. Medical students all learn the pneumonic "SLUDGE" to represent the physical findings: Salivation, Lacrimation, Urination, Defecation, Gastrointestinal upset, and Emesis. Often they remember the expanded pneumonic "SLUDGEM" to include the M for Miosis, or small pupil or muscle spasm—important considering the presentation of this case. There are other toxins which can produce some of these symptoms and signs, but few will produce all of them. For example, it is well known that opioid drugs (such as morphine, heroin, etc.) produce small pupils. One of my mentors pointed out in an article published in the early 1980s that this effect was not confined to opioids, but that even ethanol, the alcohol in liquor, can produce small pupils. SLUDGE describes the excess stimulation of certain receptors within the nervous system that are stimulated by acetylcholine, the muscarinic receptors. The muscle contractions are the result of stimulation of the nicotinic receptors. In addition to the obvious muscarinic effects, acetylcholine increases the secretion of mucous from the mucosa, or lining cells of the airways, and slows conduction of impulses through the heart. The result is excess secretions in the lungs, which can cause "internal drowning" since the secretions can so flood the airway as to be the equivalent of drowning in your own secretions, preventing oxygen from being absorbed. It can also produce a marked slowing of the heart rate. It is important to identify and distinguish between the two sets of receptors and their effects, because the treatments used targets the receptors differently. Atropine is a medication which blocks acetylcholine from attaching to the muscarinic receptor. Its administration results in the speeding up of the heart rate, drying of secretions in the lungs, and slowing down the gastrointestinal motility, thus reducing the vomiting and diarrhea.

Finding the patient having difficulty breathing, the responding paramedic intubated the patient (put a breathing tube through the patient's mouth and into the trachea, the windpipe) and ventilated him with a ball-valve bag respirator (a portable form of a mechanical ventilator). While the squad was en route to the emergency department, the staff dressed in protective gear and prepared to decontaminate the patient as soon as he arrived. The poison center staff discussed the use of atropine and the patient eventually received multiple doses of atropine both in the field as well as in the emergency department.

Fearing that the patient had ingested a nerve-agent-like pesticide, and fearing that the emergency department and its personnel might become contaminated by the patient, it was decided to decontaminate him. Today, most emergency departments have protocols for such decontamination and have special rooms and equipment in which to accomplish such decontamination without endangering either the emergency department staff or the patients. At the time of the incident, however, the emergency department did not have a separate decontamination area, so the patient was kept outside in the ambulance docking area, had his clothing removed, and then was washed down with water from a hose outside of the emergency department. Unfortunately, it was late fall and cold outside, and the only water available was cold water.

An hour later, the poison information specialist was told that the patient was now inside the emergency room. He was unresponsive, his skin was described as "warm and dry," his blood pressure was 127/56 mmHg, and his heart rate was sixty-nine beats per minute. The examination of his chest revealed bilateral rhonchi (coarse respiratory sounds, which are from fluid in the airway, sometimes called "popping in nature"), and his pupil size was reported to be three mm—smaller than when originally observed in the field. The treating team was getting ready to administer more atropine and pralidoxime. The poison information specialist discussed the doses of atropine and pralidoxime, and suggested that a naso-gastric tube be inserted to suction out any possible insecticide remaining in the patient's stomach. I was connected to the treating physician. The physician stated that nothing seemed to be helping the patient. He was still totally unresponsive and his heart rate was still low despite his having been given atropine. The decision was to give more atropine until the lungs sounded clear and then to give the pralidoxime. Pralixoxime is an agent capable of reactivating acetylcholinesterase if the binding of the enzyme to the nerve cell has not matured into a permanent bond. It works like a crow bar forcing the agent from the binding site.

The emergency department physician taking over for the next shift called the poison center an hour later; the patient's heart rate had slowed down into the 40s and the electrocardiogram revealed a wide complex arrhythmia, a very ominous finding suggesting a major defect in the normal electrical impulse propagation in the heart muscle, often associated with medications and other substances which block the normal sodium influx into the cell and can result in asystole, or stopping of the heartbeat. The arrhythmia reverted on its own to normal width. The physician told the specialist that the patient didn't really sound "wet" and that he had been given a total of 5 mg of atropine. The physician further stated that the patient had received over 7 L of intravenous fluids and had not yet produced any urine. His blood pressure was dropping and they were going to insert a central intravenous line so that they could give him more fluids as well as monitor his venous pressures. His laboratory results revealed an acidosis with a pH of 7.1 (normal 7.35–7.45), and hypokalemia with a potassium of 2.7 (normal 3.5–4.5). They found bloody mucous in his nose when trying to insert a naso-gastric (a plastic tube inserted through the nose and pushed down into the stomach, used at times to "pump the stomach") and were unsuccessful in getting the tube into his stomach. I was again conferenced in to the emergency department and discussed with the treating physician the possibility of some anti-hypertensive agent such as a calcium channel blocker or a beta blocker being ingested. Both of these medications in overdose can produce many of the clinical findings described in this case. I suggested they try administering some calcium chloride, to force calcium into his cells in case there was a calcium channel blocker involved, once the central line was in place. We also discussed the possible use of hyper-insulin euglycemia. Insulin works in several ways to increase the force of contraction of the heart and to help the peripheral vascular respond to hypotension. It has to be used in relatively high doses, and the treating team has to be careful not to let the patient's blood sugar drop too low.

The poison information specialist called back an hour later and was told that the patient's heart rate had not responded, she asked me to speak to the treating physician again. I had just arrived at my home, which was only a twenty-minute drive from the hospital. This time, I recognized real anxiety in the tone of voice of the physician. "We are going to lose this man," she stated, almost crying. "I'll be over as quickly as I can," I responded.

I arrived in the emergency department and was faced with a crowd of well-meaning healthcare providers at the bedside. They were all busy adjusting his bed, running electrocardiographs, checking his intravenous, etc. There was the constant clatter of the heart monitor and the ventilator cycling its breaths of life. I introduced myself to everyone at the bedside. After the perfunctory shaking of the hands, I walked closer to the bed. I just stood there for a moment and took the entire image in. Something seemed strange to me. The patient lay in the intensive care unit bed almost completely exposed. Often we don't think about the exposure when we are taking care of a critically ill patient; we forget the modesty element when you could miss something if you don't see all of the patient. As we soon saw, leaving this man exposed to the colder elements of the emergency room would contribute to his inability to maintain a normal body temperature. His nakedness was not what surprised me; while he was unresponsive and on a ventilator, he looked pale but pinker than I expected, considering what I had heard over the telephone. But when I touched my hand to his skin, he was "ice cold"!

Most of the time, our interest in providing medical care concerns the detection and treatment of fever or elevated body temperature. As a pediatric resident in the late 1960s, I achieved a great ability to estimate a child's temperature by placing my hand on his or her head. The normal temperature of a well person is thirty-seven degrees centigrade or ninety-eight degrees Fahrenheit. A temperature above the normal is commonly called a "fever."

Humans are mammals and, as such, are considered "warm-blooded." That means that we can maintain a constant body temperature by balancing heat production and dissipation. Cold-blooded animals maintain their body temperatures by varying their environment to effect a change. An alligator climbs out of its pond to lay on the edge in order to bake in the sun and raise its temperature. In contrast, we generally maintain a temperature above that of our surroundings by increasing heat production and decreasing heat loss when necessary.

Body heat is generated by metabolism, chemical reactions in the body which break down substrate, generally glucose, into water and carbon dioxide through various cycles or systems of metabolism. As a result of metabolism, energy, in the form of adenosine triphosphate, or ATP, is produced. ATP is then used to power other activities, such as muscle contraction and other chemical reactions. Generally these metabolic pathways aren't very efficient and there is excess heat generated in the process. There are many things which can cause an increase in body temperature. Excess muscle activity, such as in physical exertion, can lead to enough muscle contraction that there is a resultant increase in metabolic demand and production of energy, and excess heat production as a byproduct. An infection triggers the production of such excess energy, producing fever. Any imbalance of the production and loss of heat producing excess heat will result in hyperthermia. Usually this is controlled by a temperature regulating center in our brain. There is a thermal "set point," which determines when the body will respond with some adaptive mechanism to alter the internal temperature. Generally, with simple infection and simple exertion, the body's own thermoregulatory system kicks into play, and we are able to drop our temperature into a range which is safe for survival. The body loses heat through several mechanisms: the blood vessels to the skin dilate; the body becomes flushed in appearance. This so-called vasodilatation causes the detouring of blood from internal body parts closer to the surface allowing direct contact of the highly perfused hot skin to the cooler air with conduction of the heat away from the body into the air. If the air keeps moving, the conduction continues and the surface of the skin cools down. The heat can literally radiate off of the body as long as the body is not covered with some form of insulating material. In addition there may be currents of air away from the body as the result of convection produced by the hot skin surface. Additionally, evolution has provided us with the sweating mechanism. Our sweat glands release sweat onto the surface of our skin. It takes energy to convert the liquid sweat into gaseous water, the heat of vaporization. Sweat absorbs body heat and converts the liquid sweat on the surface into gaseous water vapor, and by so doing, cools the surface of the skin.

When we exert ourselves maximally or are exposed to excessive environmental temperatures, this set point may be exceeded and the temperature may overwhelm the thermoregulatory center's ability to maintain a safe body temperature. This can become an acute, life-threatening problem. Most physicians are somewhat familiar with dealing with such hyperthermia. If there is simple fever, it may not be necessary to lower the temperature; it might even be contrary to the best therapeutic intervention, since such fever may serve to starve an infectious organism. But regardless of the case, if the fever is so high that the body's mechanism to protect itself fail (so-called hyperthermia or temperature escape), then aggressive attention to decreasing the temperature as rapidly as possible, even within twenty minutes, is essential if the patient is to survive the episode. We often suggest plunging the person into an ice bath covering as much of his or her body as possible.

There is coupling of the need for energy and the production of such energy and the byproduct, heat. When uncoupled, metabolism goes wild and excess energy is produced as is heat, producing hyperthermia. There are some classic examples of substances and drugs that uncouple these reactions, resulting in hyperthermia. Dinitro-phenol, a chemical compound thought to have great potential as a weight loss product, was used to uncouple this relationship and allow a person's body temperature to rise and produce increased fat burning. The substance marketed under many names, became known as "fat burner." Unfortunately its ability to uncouple the reactions is uncontrollable and there were deaths from the resulting hyperthermia. Today other substances have been suggested as fat burners and may be found in over the counter medications or dietary supplements.

In this case, what I perceived was just the opposite. Despite the fact that his skin looked pink, it was cold to the touch. I was startled by that finding. When I asked the treating staff if they knew what his temperature was, I received no answer.

I recall them asking me, "Marcus, why are you bothering us with such a silly question? He is hypotensive, bradycardic—help us with that," were the words from one of the intensive care physicians. "Humor me," I responded, "this man is as cold as a dead fish."

In hypothermia—that is, when the body core or central temperature drops below that which is set by the internal mechanisms—metabolism slows down. Normal bodily functions decrease or stop altogether. There are animals that are capable of severely dropping their core temperature to hibernate (drop or nearly stop metabolism entirely). Man does not generally have that capability, but this patient appeared to be in just such a state. We do use induced hypothermia at times; for example, we put someone who is at risk for brain injury into such suspended animation by the use of some medications and cooling techniques. In 2015 the suggestion for patients who suffered cardiac arrest became to lower their body temperatures for at least a day, to protect their brain and provide for better recovery. Many monitoring techniques have evolved over the years to better monitor core temperatures over a wide range, but the only technique available when this gentleman presented at the hospital was the use of a standard thermometer or electronic probe.

The first thermometer they used, to humor me, was the standard electronic thermometer used in most emergency rooms and clinics at the time. It had a range from 96 to 106. You place it into the mouth or rectum of the patient and wait for a signal telling you it is time to read the temperature from a digital display. After a few moments with the probe in his rectum, the alarm sounded and the nurse stated: "His temperature is 96.5." "Isn't that the lowest that thermometer can read?" I asked. One of the other nurses answered she thought that I was correct. I asked if they had a standard rectal mercury thermometer and indeed they did. Again, when I was a resident, one of the things we had to do was to teach parents how to use a mercury thermometer, how to insert it, how long to keep it inserted and how to rotate the glass thermometer so they could see the column of mercury and read out the temperature. This was not an easy task to accomplish. But it was the standard method for assessing body temperature for more than a generation of health care providers. Today, the fear of mercury contamination has led to the abandonment of such thermometers, so most people will not be familiar with one. The nurse found one and inserted it. We waited for three or four minutes and the nurse proudly remarked: "The temperature is ninety-two degrees." Again I asked, "What is the lowest marking on the thermometer." You can guess the answer: it was ninety-two degrees.

By now I was getting a little nervous, since there are very few patients who present with such low temperatures. I had some experience with children who fell through thin ice trying to walk or skate across lakes or ponds. We simply put those children into warm clothing or a warm hot bath and they perked up, but I had rarely dealt with anyone this cold and still alive. This man weighed over a hundred kilograms, and I had no idea what we could do to actually warm him up. I did know that there was a body of scientific data to suggest that the most efficient ways was to place the victim onto a cardiac bypass machine, such as used in open-heart surgery, and to rewarm the patient "from the inside out." Thinking about that and the fact that the hospital we were now standing in had a very large cardiac surgical program, I thought that they must have a better mechanism of measuring temperatures in cold patients. We sent someone up to the operating room to borrow a temperature probe.

Shortly thereafter a triumphant aide returned from the operating room not just with a probe but with one of the cardiac surgeons who happened to be in the area and was intrigued by the story of this patient. So now there were at least 15 health care workers circling the patient in the intensive care unit. There was hardly any room to turn. The probe went into his rectum and it read twenty degrees Centigrade. We waited for it to rise; there was no change in the readout. "Holy cow," I exclaimed, "that is sixty-eight degrees Fahrenheit! I told you he felt cold." I think the staff were more impressed by my ability to rapidly convert his temperature from centigrade to Fahrenheit than the fact that I had scooped them by insisting they measure his temperature down to that range. In point of fact that was one of the very few Centigrade to Fahrenheit conversions that I can do in my head. I had done a lot of photographic work as a teenager and young adult, and all of my chemicals were used at that precise temperature, so I knew well what the conversion was. The other two points that I remember well is 0 Centigrade and 32 Fahrenheit, the temperature at which water freezes, and 212 Fahrenheit and 100 Centigrade, that at which water boils.

The staff choreographed a rapid attempt to raise his temperature. Warmed saline solution was placed into his nasogastric tube and urinary catheter. His IV fluids were warmed, and warm blankets were placed on him. They poured heated saline into every orifice in his body and even made orifices where there were no natural ones. Catheters were inserted into his chest and abdomen and warm saline instilled into those cavities as well. I was shocked at how quickly they surrounded him with their efforts to warm him up, considering the fact that I believed they had failed to recognize the severity of his problem until that instant.

"Does anyone know what medications this man is on?" I asked. "Does he have hypertension?" The only time that I have dealt with low temperatures, although not that low, was in ingestions of the antihypertensive agent clonidine, or its close cousins the imidazoline chemicals, such as that contained in over-the-counter eye drops and some nasal sprays. These medications constrict capillaries and arteries, relieving redness in the eyes and shrinking mucous membranes in both the eyes and nose through vasoconstriction. Many years before this case, we reported a series of children who drank such eye drops and presented to emergency departments unconscious, bradycardic, hypotensive, and with hypothermia, and they also had pinpoint-sized pupils, just as our patient had. When we warmed them up, their abnormal vital signs returned to normal and they awakened. There is a medication, clonidine, which has been used to treat high blood pressure (hypertension), which seems to have very similar effects.

Clonidine is a very interesting medication. Although the effects of the medication are well known, the mechanisms behind the effects are not totally clear or generally accepted. It appears to have effects on two sets of neurological receptors, and which receptor or receptors are most responsible for its therapeutic efficacy—the catecholamine receptors (often called the adrenergic receptors) or the imidazole receptors—is not universally agreed upon. The catecholamines are a group of substances which produce the symptoms recognizable as the "fight or flight" responses. They tend to be considered excitatory receptors. There are two general categories of such receptors, the alpha and the beta receptors. Medications which produce their effect by affecting such receptors are termed alpha or beta receptor agonists if they stimulate the receptor, or antagonists if they inhibit them. The alpha receptor agonists generally increase the body's responses, increasing heart rate and blood pressure. Stimulating the beta receptor increases the force of contraction of the heart muscle and dilates the bronchial tree. The beta receptor is also involved with the breakdown of glycogen, an energy source derived from glucose and stored in the liver for reconversion back to glucose when needed. When a medication which has alpha agonist activity is administered to a patient, the expected results are hypertension and tachycardia. Clonidine, an alpha receptor agonist, works centrally, at the presynaptic junction, to stimulate the central alpha receptor. Clonidine appears to have greater affinity for the alpha 2 receptor. It is thought that binding centrally causes the decrease in cytoplasmic calcium levels and thus decreases the sympathetic outflow from the brain and results in the hypothermia, hypotension, and bradycardia. This in turn interferes with the feedback loop, "fooling" the brain into thinking there is more catecholamine in the blood then there is. Thus, stimulation of this receptor decreases the peripheral vascular tone, decreases peripheral resistance and results in vasodilatation, hypotension and bradycardia. It also effects thermoregulation centrally and because of the peripheral vasodilatation increases the loss of heat from the skin.

There is also evidence that clonidine may produce some of its effects via stimulation of the imidazole receptors. As with the catecholamine receptors, there are several imidazole receptors. The imidazole-1 receptor, like the alpha-2 catecholamine receptor, seems to be located centrally, within the brain. It has been shown to be involved in the cardiovascular effects of clonidine. One hypothesis is that clonidine's effects are somehow caused by some combination or interaction, perhaps a sequential effect of both the alpha-2 and imidazole receptor action.

I did not know that sometime before I got to the hospital, a call was made to the patient's primary-care physician asking him if he could shed some light on the man's past medical history. While the team was in the process of warming the patient up, the physician arrived with a copy of the patient's medical record. The physician explained that yes, the patient had a history of hypertension, and yes he was receiving clonidine as one of the agents to treat his hypertension.

The clinical picture of the patient now was that of the toxidrome associated with clonidine or a clonidine-like substance. There was a history of access to the medication. We only had to wait until the patient regained consciousness to ask whether he took an overdose. Over the next six to eight hours, his temperature rose to normal and his blood pressure and heart rate also responded and rose to normal. Upon awakening, he expressed the fact that he was despondent over the loss of his wife and had, yes, taken an overdose of the clonidine.

After recovery from the overdose, he was transferred to an in-patient psychiatric facility for a few days and then discharged to his family. There were no apparent medical complications of his overdose.

Generally speaking, hypothermia is not as acutely life-threatening a problem as is hyperthermia. Evolution has afforded us better mechanisms to deal with hypothermia than hyperthermia. There is a much lower tolerance for elevated body temperatures than for lower temperatures. There is the risk of abnormal cardiac rhythm at temperatures in the low to middle nineties, although that toxicity doesn't hold a candle to the effects of prolonged hyperthermia, which can literally "cook" the proteins in the brain and cause the demise of the patient. Hypothermia, in contrast, rarely produces enough tissue damage to compare it to hyperthermia.

Suggested Reading

Head GA, Chan CKS, Burke SL. Relationship between imidazoline and alpha2-adrenoreceptors involved in the sympatho-inhinitory actions of centrally acting antihypertensive agents. J Auton Nerv Syst. 1998;72:163–9.

Szabo B. Imidasoline antihypertensice drugs: a critical review on their mechanism of action. Pharmacol Ther. 2002;93(1):931–5.

Chapter 4
The Pig from North Jersey

The telephone rang one morning and it was Peri Kamalakar, a physician who specialized in pediatric hematology. I met Peri in 1972, when I first came to New Jersey as a young attending pediatrician. I was the director of the pediatric clinic and Peri was the pediatric chief resident. He went on to study pediatric hematology and oncology and returned to the hospital years later as its pediatric hematologist. He had a patient that he wanted to discuss with me. The child was one of a set of twins that he was seeing for anemia (the child's hemoglobin was 8.2 g/dL with a normal of over 11), referred by her pediatrician. The child in question had a low mean cell volume (MCV, a measurement of the size of a red blood cell with a normal of 70–100 fL) The child's MCV was 50 fL, and she also had a low mean cell hemoglobin concentration (MCH, a measure of the concentration of hemoglobin, the oxygen carrying molecule, inside each red blood cell). This combination is commonly seen in iron deficiency, a common problem in small, rapidly growing children whose diets are frequently insufficient in iron. He had treated the child for iron deficiency thinking that the child had iron deficiency and thalassemia minor, a not uncommon inherited abnormality of hemoglobin formation seen in many individuals with ethnic origins in the greater Mediterranean basin (this child was ethnically an Italian American). Interestingly, he thought to draw a blood lead level and found that the lead level was elevated, 37 mcg/dL, which is in the moderately elevated range. (In 2012 the United States Centers for Disease Control and Prevention set a "reference level" for childhood blood lead levels at the top 2.5% of the population, or at that time 5 mcg/dL.) His call was to determine what I would suggest to do about the elevation in the lead level. I suggested that the treatment for iron deficiency continue and that he coordinate an investigation be initiated by the local health department in an effort to find the source of lead-exposure and to eliminate it. I further suggested that the lead level be watched to see if it might drop with the rise in the child's iron and hemoglobin. Three months later, in August, his office called and told me that the child's lead level was now 42 mcg/dL and I suggested hospitalization. Such an approach, I explained, would enable us to treat the child, lowering her lead level while separating her from any possible source of further lead exposure. During her

© Springer International Publishing AG 2017
S.M. Marcus, *Medical Toxicology: Antidotes and Anecdotes*,
DOI 10.1007/978-3-319-51029-3_4

hospitalization the public health officials could do their sleuthing, to determine the exposure source and eliminate it. The basic tenet of treatment of lead poisoning is to find the source or sources of exposure and to eliminate it/them. Medical therapy with medication is considered only as adjunctive therapy to the removal from the source.

The child was subsequently admitted. I was called to see her when she arrived. I spoke to the family and the father stated that they had antique painted furniture in the home and that the paint on the furniture was peeling. He thought that might have been the cause. The father also stated that he just replaced doors in the house so perhaps the child was exposed to lead in the paint on the doors. The parents reported that the child drank large amounts of milk. They were told by Dr. Kamalakar, as part of the treatment for the iron deficiency, that they needed to cut down on the amount of milk the child was consuming. They were also diluting the milk to decrease the ingestion of milk because of the iron deficiency that was being treated by hematology. That dietary manipulation makes sense for the iron deficiency, since milk does seem to interfere with the absorption of iron, and some individuals actually lose blood, and thus iron, in their stools from drinking too much milk. Unfortunately, if one does not have enough calcium in one's diet, and is exposed to any lead through the gastrointestinal tract, the lead is maximally absorbed. In addition, iron deficiency has the effect of "turning on" a gene in the cells in the small intestine that absorb metal ions, such as iron and calcium, but with the absence of those ions, the cells absorb lead. We obtained an abdominal X-ray which showed no recent ingestion of any radiopaque material (lead-containing paint chips show up as radiopaque foreign bodies on an X-ray).

I called the local health department to find out if they had found any source of lead that the child might have had access to and might have ingested. The health officer said that they found "tooth marks" on the windowsills in the home. The paint on the windowsills tested positive for lead. The child was started on oral chelation therapy with succimer in the hospital. The term *chelation* is derived from the Greek *chele*, or "claw," for the parts of the molecule which bind the lead and are arranged around the molecule like the legs of a crab, binding the lead and thereby deactivating its toxicity. There are other chelators that can be used, but this one can be taken orally. This medication has approval from the United States Food and Drug Administration to be used in children with blood lead levels above 45 µg per deciliter of blood. This awful smelling and tasting medication is absorbed from the intestines and binds with lead in the bloodstream, enabling the lead to be passed in the stool and urine of the patient. The medication is available in capsule form, which must be diluted in applesauce or other non-dairy food since small children do not swallow capsules. The smell and taste particularly in this format is often not well tolerated. The treatment team was lucky this time, as the child tolerated the therapy very well and was discharged from the hospital on oral succimer chelation therapy.

After discharge from the hospital, I continued to see the child and her family in my office to monitor her recovery from lead poisoning. At the end of chelation therapy, her blood lead level had dropped into the teens. Her hemoglobin rose to thirteen and a half grams per deciliter and her MCV to 71. While in the hospital I noted that her blood work showed an interesting finding: an abundance of eosinophils, a type of white blood cell frequently seen in individuals with allergies. Having seen it before in lead poisoned individuals, I did not make much of it at the time and felt I would simply monitor it as she recovered from both her iron deficiency and lead poisoning. On follow-up, the laboratory continued to report elevations in eosinophils. The quantity of these cells is generally reported by the laboratory in either percentage of white cells, and her eosinophil count was 10% (normally less than 3%), or in terms of absolute number of such cells (multiply the percentage by the total number of white cells). In her case, although the percentage was initially high, the total "absolute" number of eosinophils was in the normal range.

In following the course of the child's chelation and monitoring her progress as to possible re-exposure, her eosinophil count remained elevated, both in percentage and total number as well. The persistence of the elevated eosinophil count (eosinophilia) led me to look for possible causes of the elevated eosinophil count. Allergic reactions are frequently associated with eosinophilia, but I found nothing to suggest an allergic reaction. Another cause of eosinophilia is intestinal parasite infestations. Humans often develop parasitic infestations from contact with infested pets. I learned that although the family had no pets, their neighbors had puppies that the child liked to play with. There seemed to be no obvious allergic reaction to the pets, but we were concerned that perhaps the puppies might be a source of exposure to worms. Since it was possible that the child could have become infested with intestinal roundworms, we suggested that the neighbors have their dogs checked. The family learned from the neighbors that, in fact, their dogs did have worms and they were treated by their veterinarian. This prompted me to attempt to determine if the child might have an intestinal infestation of worms. There was difficulty getting the child tested for parasitic infestation. The normal test is to examine stools for ova (eggs) released by parasites into the intestines. We asked the family to collect three samples of stool and then submit the samples to a laboratory for investigation. That turned out to be no easy task. I must not have described the collection process clearly enough, since the parents simply divided one stool into thirds. We wanted them to collect three different stools at different times to increase the likelihood that, if the child was infested, we would find evidence of the parasite in at least one of the samples. When the family finally accomplished the appropriate stool collection, testing showed no sign of parasitic infestation.

The eosinophilia kept nagging me. I asked for the records of her previous blood tests and noticed that from the initial examination at the hematologist's office, her eosinophil count was consistently elevated. This was discussed with the family and continued to be a subject of concern on subsequent visits to the office while I was tracking her lead exposure.

Many years before this case, I became interested in the association of eosinophilia and lead poisoning. I reached out to Dr. Julian Chisholm, the major guru of lead poisoning at the time, and found that over many years of his involvement with children with lead poisoning, it was not uncommon to see eosinophilia associated with lead poisoning. He and I discussed this curious finding but were unable to explain it. About a decade before the child we were now treating, a child was admitted to the same hospital as this patient for lead poisoning, and while in the hospital developed a seizure despite having a level of lead that normally would not be expected to result in a seizure. The infectious disease service was consulted for the possibility of an infection-related seizure. The child's white blood cell count revealed an elevated eosinophil count. As I stated previously, these cells are elevated with allergy or when an individual is recovering from some illnesses or has a parasitic infection. The consulting infectious disease physician postulated that the child might have an intestinal parasite infestation associated with seizures called visceral larva migrans (VLM). That index case started me on a course of investigation. One of the pediatric residents (twenty years later to become the Director of Pediatrics at that hospital), and I found that almost 25% of the children I treated for lead poisoning had serological evidence of infection with ascariasis, a common roundworm infestation that produces VLM which is in turn, often associated with eosinophilia. Visceral larva migrans is a condition caused by worms, generally Toxocara, a common worm that infects the intestines of dogs and cats. The dog parasite is called *Toxocara canis* and the cat parasite is called *Toxocara cati*. Eggs produced by these worms within the intestines of the cat or dog are passed into the feces of the infected animals. Outbreaks have occurred in the United States in children who play in areas with soil contaminated by dog or cat feces. Young children with pica (the habit of eating nonfood substances; in children with lead poisoning, often lead-based paint) are at highest risk. In our study of lead poisoned children with eosinophilia and lead poisoning, there were often dogs or cats in the homes that were frequently allowed to defecate in the same backyard where the children played. It was our belief that eggs in the dog feces contaminated the soil in their backyards, and the children were exposed from putting their dirty hands in their mouths (the United States Environmental Protection Agency has stated that the average toddler ingests 200–400 mg of soil each day) or from eating with their hands without adequately washing hands between playing in the yard and eating. After a person swallows the worm eggs, the eggs hatch in the gastrointestinal tract and are carried throughout the body to various organs, such as the lungs, liver, and eyes. The brain, heart, and other organs can also be affected. At times, the movement of the worms throughout the brain triggers seizures. There are times where live worms are seen in the stool, usually to the horror of the observer, parent or hospital nurse.

The testing for that previous study was done as a favor to me by someone at the Centers for Disease Control (CDC). Reflecting on those cases and this current child, I reached out to the CDC to see if they could provide serological testing for the child. I could not find anybody at the CDC whom I had worked with the past, so this issue was pushed to my "back burner."

About five months after the child was initially hospitalized, in January, I read an article in the *Journal of the American Medical Association* about the presentation of a patient from South America at Johns Hopkins Hospital with eosinophilia, and, as in our case, the patient was asymptomatic. The paper, authored by Kathleen Page, M.D., discussed various parasitic causes of asymptomatic eosinophilia and included the statement that "patients with an absolute eosinophil count of more than 3000/µL or more than 1500/µL for more than six months are at risk of end organ damage and should be referred for specialized parasitic and/or hematological consultation."

Included in the article was a suggested workup for a patient with unknown eosino-philia. It contained a caveat that using a commercial laboratory rather than the CDC might produce spurious results. This article revived my interest in the possibility that this child might be infected with some parasite. At that time, my daughter, Leigh, was a fellow in pediatric hematology and oncology at the Johns Hopkins Hospital and I asked that she reach out to Dr. Page and see whether I might contact her to discuss my case. After confirming a contact number and her willingness to discuss the case, I called Dr. Page. We had a lengthy conversation about how to pursue the investigation of this child. She gave me the name of a person at the CDC and suggested I call and use her name as a referral source.

I contacted Dr. LeAnne Fox at the CDC and discussed the case with her. Dr. Fox agreed to get involved in my efforts to establish a cause of this child's eosinophilia. She had not known of my work on VLM, but was interested and agreed to have the CDC's lab do the testing for my patient. A blood specimen was submitted by me to the CDC in late February, six months after her hospitalization for lead poisoning (I was later to discover that submitting a specimen directly to the CDC and not through the proper channels was discouraged). The CDC laboratory did a serological test for toxacara, the worm responsible for this infestation, and found no evidence of such an infestation. In discussions with Dr. Fox, she informed me that her laboratory was setting up a serological test for strongyloides, the next likely culprit as per her dis-cussion. Strongyloides, commonly called threadworm, is another worm that has been implicated in human intestinal infestations. This worm is not common in developed countries and has a complex life cycle. The infection is often asymptom-atic. The worm generally infects a human when exposed to the larvae of the worm through the skin. This can occur from entering contaminated water or contact with larvae in the soil. Like Toxacara, strongyloides are often found in pets. Once the larvae enter the body through the skin, they mature and travel throughout the body, sometimes reaching the lung, where they can be coughed up and swallowed and the individual then becomes auto-infected. The infection is associated with eosino-philia. I did explain that the child's stools were examined and were negative for any ova, and she stated that the serological test would be a more sensitive test. Dr. Fox said that serological testing would be done just as soon as the testing became vali-dated. A month later Dr. Fox informed me that that the strongyloides testing was negative, and we had another lengthy discussion since the child's eosinophil count was still elevated. She told me that she would think about what else to do and would do follow-up testing. She still had the blood I sent to her, so there was no need for further sampling.

A month later, in late April, I received an email from the infectious disease prac-titioner at the hospital, a nurse who coordinates the care and follow-up of cases of infectious diseases at the hospital. She explained that she received notification from the New Jersey State Department of Health and Senior Services (NJDHSS) of a posi-tive test for Trichinella, a pork parasite, on a patient thought by the state to have been to the hospital. She couldn't find that patient registered at the hospital and for some reason she wondered if I knew anything about the patient. To say the least, I was amazed that this result went through such a convoluted path to get to me, particularly since I had not heard anything directly from the CDC. I immediately contacted Dr. Fox and she confirmed the result. I was forwarded a copy of the result from the February blood test which was officially reported as negative for strongyloides; further, the blood had a titer of 1:2 for toxocara canis (VLM), which is considered as negative (positive is greater than 1:32 with specificity of 90%), but a serological test for trichinella of 2.3010, with anything above 0.4 as being considered positive with specificity of 95%. When she confirmed this finding, we arranged to have another specimen sent to her laboratory, and to sample the other family members as well. In attempting the follow-up, I discovered that I had violated procedure by going directly to the CDC and not through the New Jersey Department of Health and Senior Services (NJDHSS, subsequently renamed the New Jersey Department of Health). It is an interesting "catch 22" that although a physician is within his or her right to ask the CDC to help with an individual patient, and in such a case the CDC can act as a reference laboratory, it is more common for a physician to ask for the involvement of his or her local health department and for that department in turn to ask for CDC involvement if deemed necessary. Although NJDHSS's laboratory was unable to do the testing needed, and had to send the specimens to the CDC to do additional testing, I had to fill out all of the forms for submission to NJDHSS and to send them to NJDHSS. Upon receipt in NJDHSS' laboratory, they re-wrapped the specimens and forwarded them to the CDC. I was concerned about both the delay in processing and the possibility of error in marking the specimens, loss of specimen or their damage, but was assured by NJDHSS that they would do the processing appropriately and in a timely fashion.

I then drew a repeat blood test on this child, as well as blood from her twin sister and her parents. The repeat blood test on this child was reported as 2.7630, a rise in serological titer. Her sister's blood test was also found to be elevated at a level of 2.7970. Interestingly, neither parent tested positive, her father tested at 0.3540 and her mother at 0.1610.

These findings led to further questioning of the family to see if we could find a common source for the exposure of the two children which would have occurred while not exposing the parents. In discussion with the parents it was determined that the maternal grandmother had died the summer before and the children spent a lot of time with the paternal grandmother. This elderly Italian woman made meatballs and meat sauce that the girls loved to eat. The grandmother made typical "Italian meatballs." They were made from three meats: ground beef, veal and pork. This woman had been hospitalized for three days with diarrhea and dehydration and there was no cause ever determined. The exact timing was unclear as to when she was hospitalized and when the girls were first found to have eosinophilia. Both children and the grandmother were totally asymptomatic at the time the serological tests of the children were reported as positive.

I tried to get the grandmother tested. Asking her to submit to blood testing resulted in a bit of a family feud. The parents explained that the grandmother was upset; "how can you think that I would have poisoned the girls?" was apparently her response to their questions and request for a blood test. This went on for weeks, causing much family tension. Finally she agreed but, for some unexplained reason, would not allow us to send the blood to the CDC, so it was sent to a commercial laboratory, and the results were negative. Unfortunately, the serological testing for trichinella is not a standard test and it is unknown if the test used by the laboratory her physician sent the test to had the sensitivity and specificity of the test the CDC used. It is also possible, since the titers in an affected individual eventually fall, that it was too late to confirm her infection. Thus, it may have been a false negative.

Trichinellosis (also sometimes called trichinosis) is the clinical disease caused by the round worm trichinella. Trichinella are the smallest round worm (nematode) parasite of humans and are one of the most widespread and clinically important parasites in the world. Infection with this worm can produce serious morbidity and even mortality. The infection occurs when someone eats undercooked meat containing larvae of the parasitic worm *Trichinella spiralis*. Evidence of the existence of the parasite has been genetically dated to 1000 million years ago. Today, species of the genus trichinella inhabit virtually the entire surface of the globe. The larvae are found in various meats, including pork products, wild boar, bear, walrus, and other carnivorous game.

The existence of infection with the worm was not uncommon in the United States up to and during the 1940s, there were 500 cases reported each year. Two postmortem studies, reported in two different geographical areas of the United States in the 1940s, found the prevalence rate (the number of cases present in a certain population; this is different from incidence, which is just the number of new cases) to be 15–20%. The number of reported cases per year in the United States has declined since the CDC first began collecting statistics in 1947. In the period 1977–1981, the average number of reported cases per year was 137. In 1982–1986, this figure dropped to 57 cases. The incidence continued to drop and, except for a slight spike in reported cases in 2008, the annual number of reported cases in the United States remains in the teens. No apparent change in the surveillance system can account for this downward trend. Although infected pork continues to be the main source of human infection, the decline in the annual incidence of trichinosis over the last twelve years appears to be due to a decrease in cases traceable to commercial pork products. The absolute number of cases attributed annually to wild animal sources, such as wild boar, bear, and other carnivorous game, has remained relatively constant since 1975. In Eastern Europe the incidence is higher. For example, in 2004 there were 780 cases reported in Romania. During the years in which there were appreciable numbers of cases reported in the United States, there was a consistent seasonal pattern for trichinosis, with a peak in December and January. This was thought to be related to the consumption of homemade pork sausage during the Christmas holidays. In 1986, 25 cases (49%) were reported in December and January. Of the eleven cases reported for January, four were traced to a common-source outbreak associated with homemade pork sausage in Massachusetts. The pork used to prepare this sausage came directly from a small farm. Five additional cases were traced to a common-source outbreak associated with wild boar in New Hampshire. Of the 14 cases reported in December, 12 were traced to a common-source outbreak associated with ingestion of bear meat in Pennsylvania.

The cause of the decrease in reported cases is unclear. Several activities at the national and state level have improved prospects for the control and prevention of trichinosis in commercial pork products. The Federal Swine Health Protection Act (Public Law 96-468) of October 17, 1980, specifically prohibits the feeding of food waste products to swine unless the garbage is treated to kill disease-causing organisms, including *T. spiralis*. Enforcement of the act is the joint responsibility of the individual states and of the U.S. Department of Agriculture's (USDA's) Animal and Plant Health Inspection Service (APHIS). The National Pork Producers Council (NPPC), in cooperation with the USDA, developed a rapid enzyme-linked immunosorbent assay (ELISA) test to detect hogs with trichinosis before slaughter. The NPPC and USDA actively promote hog-management practices that avoid factors epidemiologically linked to the transmission of trichinosis. They require the immediate removal of dead hogs from feed lots, effective rat control, and other methods that eliminate the interaction of commercial hogs and wild animals.

The best estimate of the overall prevalence of trichinosis in marketed hogs in the United States is 0.1%. This estimate is based on a study of farm-raised butchered hogs for 1966–1970. There may be a wide variation in trichinella-contamination based on geography. Infection seems to be more common in colder climates. In a slaughterhouse-based survey of 1223 hogs in Louisiana, only one (less than 0.1%) infected animal was detected. No infection was found among 3245 hogs from slaughterhouses in Minnesota, Wisconsin, Iowa, South Dakota, and North Dakota examined from 1983 to 1985. The animals examined were from both small family farms where pigs were raised for home consumption and from large commercial operations.

Despite the lower prevalence of contaminated pork, the continued role of public education concerning the proper cooking of pork to eliminate the risk of trichinosis cannot be overstated. Whereas commercial pork products are declining as a cause of trichinosis, noncommercial sources of pork—such as small farms not using modern hog-management practices—and wild animal meats are emerging as important sources of human trichinosis in the United States. People who buy pork from small farms or who eat wild animal meats should be educated as to how to eliminate their risk of acquiring trichinosis.

People acquire trichinellosis by consuming raw or undercooked meat infected with the *Trichinella* parasite, particularly wild game meat (for example, bear meat) or pork. Even tasting very small amounts of uncooked or undercooked meat during preparation or cooking puts you at risk for infection. Outbreaks occur in settings where multiple people consume the same *Trichinella*-infected meat.

The life cycle of the worm begins when an animal host ingests meat containing encapsulated larvae. Digestion of the cystic capsule by intestinal juices releases larvae which then pass into the small intestine, where they invade the epithelium (internal lining) of the intestines. The larvae grow and molt eventually maturing into adult sexual forms. The adult forms then pass into the intestinal lumen where they mate. The female worms then burrow back into the intestinal wall and release new larvae, up to 1500 per female worm, before the host's immunological system expels the adult worms. The newborn larvae then migrate through the intestinal wall into the blood stream and are carried throughout the body eventually making their way into the capillaries of muscles in which they become encysted. If the host is a pig and the parasite becomes encysted in muscle and humans eat the meat, the worm life cycle repeats itself, this time in the human. The human, on the top of the food chain, represents the end of the cycle.

Clinical disease consists of several stages. The first occurs within twelve hours to two days after the ingestion of meat contaminated with cysts (aka nurse cells) and symptoms consist of nausea and diarrhea, usually mild. With the maturation of the larval form into adults and invasion of the intestinal mucosa, upper gastrointestinal pain, malaise, and low-grade fever may be found. After a few weeks, the intestinal stage of the infestation ceases and the parenteral phase begins with the migration of larvae throughout the body. The result may be diffuse muscle pain (myalgia), swelling of the face (edema), particularly around the eyes, red eyes (conjunctivitis), fever, headache, skin rash, and other symptoms. Generally, although muscles are the end organs damaged, the heart muscle is spared. Occasionally inflammation of the heart and brain does occur and is likely the cause of the rare mortality seen. The host body's response to the invasion by the worms includes the production of the white cell eosinophil, as seen in the twins.

The preferred means of diagnosis is the examination of infected muscle. If there is localized muscle involvement, a muscle biopsy and examination under the microscope will reveal the encapsulated cysts. Since the use of muscle biopsy represents some risk, an alternate methodology, an enzyme-linked immunosorbent assay (ELISA), can be used, and this was the case for these girls. ELISA combined with confirmatory western blot testing, has become a standard in the surveillance programs to monitor the spread of the worm in swine herds. ELISA detectable antibodies peak in the second or third month post infection and then gradually decline, but may remain positive for years.

Treatment is most often symptomatic and supportive, with pain medication and anti-inflammatory agents such as ibuprofen. In more serious cases, treatment may include mebendazole or albendazole. Generally, treatment is most effective during the gastrointestinal phase and is less useful once the encysting phase has begun. Both anti-helminths are considered safe but have been associated with suppression of bone-marrow production.

The patient remained asymptomatic as both her lead level and eosinophil levels dropped to normal over the next two years.

Suggested Reading

Blaga R, Durand B, Antoniu S, et al. A dramatic increase in the incidence of human trichinellosis in Romania over the past 25 years: impact of political changhes and regional food habits. Am J Trop Med. 2007;76(5):983–6.

International Commission on Trichinellosis: run international conferences every year the abstracts and presentations are available through the commissions website: http://www.trichinellosis. org/Conferences.php.

Page KR, Zenilman J. Eosinophilia in a patient from South America. JAMA. 2008;299(4):437–44.

Chapter 5
Murder in the ICU

It all began innocently on the afternoon of June 18, 2003.[1] Shirley Rendon was the poison information specialist on duty at the New Jersey Poison Center (also known as the New Jersey Poison Information and Education System, NJPIES), which was then located in its temporary quarters in the Stanley Bergen Building at University of Medicine and Dentistry of New Jersey in Newark. These were quarters shared with Newark's Emergency Medical Services Medical Dispatch Center, a rather dark and depressing work area at the time. Shirley was a physician trained in medical school in the Dominican Republic. By her experience and ability to pass a national certification examination, she was certified as a Specialist in Poison Information by the American Association of Poison Control Centers.

The call was made by a nurse practitioner, Mary Kelly. She was calling about a forty-year-old Asian woman who had been admitted to Somerset Medical Center with a history of a cancer, T-cell lymphoma, and cardiomyopathy. Lymphomas consist of several cancers affecting the lymphatic system. They can be confined to lymph tissues, such as lymph nodes, but some spread into the circulation, acting like leukemias. Lymphatic cells are either T cell or B cells. T-cell lymphomas represent about 10% of all lymphomas. The medications used to treat these cancers are known to produce damage to heart muscle and it was believed that her myocardiopathy, heart damage, was probably the side effect of the treatments she had received for her cancer. She was admitted to the hospital to receive a blood transfusion and to evaluate her rapid heart rate. Prior to her admission to the hospital, she was receiving the medication digoxin, a drug long used to slow heart rate and help strengthen the heart, in an effort to help her cardiomyopathy. Digoxin in proper dosage will slow

---

[1] All quotations from printed material (correspondence, newspaper articles, and press releases) are direct quotations. All dialogue is derived from conversations recorded by the Poison Center or from notes made contemporaneously and included on electronic records stored in the archives of the center.

© Springer International Publishing AG 2017
S.M. Marcus, *Medical Toxicology: Antidotes and Anecdotes*,
DOI 10.1007/978-3-319-51029-3_5

down the heart rate and increase the force of the muscle contraction. On June 13, the medication was discontinued because of an abnormality observed on her electrocardiogram. A cardiology consultant felt that she had "sick sinus syndrome." The "sinus" is the part of the heart that originates the electrical discharge which produces the organized contraction of the heart. If it becomes damaged, "sick," it may slow or fail to initiate such an impulse and hence slow the heart. To avoid complicating the issue with the drug, the cardiologist ordered that the digoxin be discontinued. Three days later, while allegedly no longer taking the digoxin, the patient developed a severe slowing of her heart rate. A digoxin level was obtained and the results startled the staff. The blood test result showed a high level of digoxin, 9.3 ng/mL (normally an effective level would be in the range of 1.5 ng/mL). Over the next few days her level dropped to 2.36 ng/mL—the level at the time of the call to NJPIES.

The caller stated that they checked to be sure no further digoxin was given to the patient, and found no record of such. The staff had asked the family if there was anything that they may have brought in that might be implicated, thinking about some herbal or folk remedy. As it turned out, the patient was drinking a tea made from the bark of a mulberry tree and mushrooms. They supplied the staff at Somerset with the names of the mushrooms: *Phellinus linteus* aoshima, *Phellinus igniarius* quell, *Phellinus yucatensis* imazk, *Phellinus yucatensis* murr, and *Phellinus yucatensis* pyropolyrous. Mary was interested in learning if any of these mushrooms could cause an increase in the patient's digoxin level. I was "conferenced" into the call and stated that I did not know of any mushroom that contained anything like digoxin but that there are other products which do. I suggested that they review the electrocardiograms and laboratory data from the time of her admission, and if there was blood left from any of the days prior to June 16, that the blood be tested for digoxin. I asked Mary to send us all of the laboratory data, a summary of the case, and some of the mushrooms. We said that we would research the mushroom names and try to find someone to analyze them. I also suggested that they check their assay and be sure that their laboratory was confident with the results. Bruce Ruck, Pharm.D., the director of drug information at the poison center, also jumped into the call and suggested they try to recreate the tea that she drank so that we could try to measure digoxin-like substances in it.

We assigned the chore of looking up the mushrooms listed by the family to a pharmacy student who was rotating with us as part of her drug information and toxicology experience as a student at the Rutgers College of Pharmacy. We also contacted the group of mycologists, experts in identification of mushrooms, who work as consultants to the poison center to help us identify toxic mushrooms. The five mushrooms, all members of the same genus, are so similar as to say they are essentially the same. The mushroom does in fact grow on the trunk bark of the mulberry tree, hence the comment by the family that the tea is mulberry tea. The tea is said to enhance the immune system, to help overcome cancer, and to be an indirect treatment of geriatric disease. The mycologists drew a blank on the question of mushrooms containing anything like the drug digoxin. The pharmacy student was unable to find any evidence that it would interfere with a digoxin assay.

Bruce and I spoke about the situation and wondered if digoxin levels could reach that high from an interaction with antibiotics. It is known that there is considerable metabolism of digoxin within the intestines by bacteria, which tends to decrease the absorption of orally administered digoxin. Thus when a patient ingests some antibiotics, the absorption may rise, occasionally resulting in a very high digoxin level. It did not seem to us that one could expect the level to rise to the extent it did in this patient, and the fact that we were told that she was not receiving any digoxin would suggest that this was not part of the situation. We also considered the possibility of the production of digoxin-like substances by the patient's body. This has been reported in some cases of liver disease, in which a substance which has effects like digoxin, and can at times be measured, can be found. Again, we could not find any evidence of levels anywhere near that of this patient. When Richard Casas, one of the other information specialists, called the hospital to report our efforts at researching the mushrooms, Mary Kelly was unavailable but Casas was able to discuss our findings with a resident physician and learned that the patient was not receiving any antibiotics.

On June 25, Shirley Rendon was able to reach Mary Kelly and relayed our findings regarding the mushrooms. In turn, Rendon learned that the patient was much better clinically and her digoxin level was now very low. She sent us a letter with information about the case. She included in the package a sample of the mushroom mix the family provided for analysis. Her letter stated that "on June 13th the patient experienced a six second pause of heart beat. Cardiology evaluated her and made the diagnosis of 'sick sinus syndrome.'" She had been on digoxin and it was stopped that day, her last dose was 0.125 mg. On June 16th she was found to be bradycardic (had a low heart rate) and her digoxin level was found to be 9.3 ng/mL. The patient and family were questioned about any medications she may have used as well as any herbal and home remedies. That is how the question of mushrooms arose. She stated that at our suggestion they tested stored serum from admission and the digoxin level was "normal."

On July 3, I brought the mushrooms to a New York City Poison Center's Consultant's Conference, a monthly meeting organized by the staff of the New York City Poison Center in the conference room at the New York City Department of Health building on First Avenue in Manhattan. Participants at these sessions consist of emergency room physicians and toxicologists from the greater New York City area, often from as far as Massachusetts and Texas. The cases presented for discussion at the conference are often presented as unknown poisonings, with only preliminary information. It affords the opportunity to tap into the combined experience of a large number of clinicians. I didn't present the case that day, but did ask if anyone had ever heard of any mushrooms with cardiac glycoside action, or any which might cause a false positive digoxin level. No one said that they had. Robert Hoffman, M.D., the director of New York City's Poison Center, said that he would get someone to analyze the mushrooms for us.

The following week, on July 8, Nancy, one of the pharmacists from the pharmacy at Somerset Medical Center, called the poison center. She spoke to information specialist Ralph Lucanie, a pharmacist with many years of experience at another poison center before transferring to ours. She stated that she was asked by a hospital "sentinel event team" to calculate the amount of digoxin someone would have to take to bump his digoxin level from 1.33 to 9.61 in one day. A "sentinel event" is defined by the United States Joint Commission on Hospital Accreditation, the certifying body for hospital accreditation, as an unexpected occurrence involving death or serious physical or psychological injury, or the risk thereof. Serious injury specifically includes loss of limb or function. The phrase, "or the risk thereof" includes any process variation for which a recurrence would carry a significant chance of a serious adverse outcome. Such events are called "sentinel" because they signal the need for immediate investigation and response.

She stated that she was involved in a "sentinel event" investigation about an elderly patient in their ICU with multiple organ failure and on dialysis. She mentioned that a few weeks ago her hospital had reached out to us regarding a patient in their unit who developed digoxin toxicity and there was a question about mushrooms, but now this second patient developed digoxin toxicity and died. Neither Bruce Ruck nor I was available at the time, so Ralph took her telephone number and said that he would have Bruce call her back.

When Bruce called the pharmacist back, he told her that we were getting the mushroom from the prior case analyzed. He thought the first case had an elevated digoxin level toxic on admission.

"No, she did not!" Nancy clarified that the first victim, the woman who drank the mushrooms tea, was taking digoxin and mushroom tea at home and was not digoxin toxic on admission. In fact, when she became toxic, the hospital analyzed her first blood from admission and it was "okay."

The pharmacist explained that now they had a sixty-eight-year-old man who came in with pneumonia on June 13. He had a very complicated medical problem with Idiopathic thrombocytopenic purpura (an unexplained drop in his platelets leading to bleeding in his skin, which gave a characteristic bruised appearance to the skin, which is technically called purpura), hypertension, hypothyroidism, a history of Coronary Artery Bypass Graft surgery, and diabetes mellitus. While in the hospital, he developed atrial fibrillation (a rapid heartbeat in the upper chamber of the heart—a very common arrhythmia). The treating team gave him synthroid (thyroid hormone) by injection and started him on amiodarone (a drug to slow down the heart) for the atrial fibrillation. He was on amiodarone in an intravenous drip from June 14 to June 20. He subsequently developed kidney and liver failure. On June 19 he received two doses of digoxin 0.25 mg and had daily renal dialysis for his kidney failure from June 15 on. She stated that the hospital staff monitored his digoxin level. On June 20 he was found to have a level of 1.2 ng/mL, on June 22 it was 1.08. He received another dose of digoxin on June 24, of 0.125 mg, then had levels on June 26 of 1.59 ng/mL and on June 27 1.33 ng/mL. On June 28 his digoxin level suddenly rose to 9.61 ng/mL and he developed cardiac arrest. He was administered antidotal therapy, a drug called Digibind, which is an antibody produced in sheep that, when injected into a digoxin-toxin patient, binds to the digoxin circulation in the blood thereby deactivating it, and reversing toxicity. Often, depending on how the level is measured after the antibody is administered, the level will seem to rise. Indeed, a repeat digoxin level after the antibody was determined to be 21, not unexpected since the assay measures the digoxin bound to the antibody as well as that which circulates free of the antibody.

Bruce said that this could only be lab error, or someone gave him digoxin. He questioned the intravenous synthroid. Could that have been digoxin by error? The pharmacist stated that the pharmacy sends synthroid up in a box, and it is not obtained from the pixus, a medication dispensing device on most hospital units which is stocked with a variety of commonly used medications.

Bruce discussed the effect on clearance of digoxin by amiodarone. Digoxin is generally cleared (eliminated) by the kidneys. If the kidneys fail to work properly, digoxin will not be cleared by the body. He explained that the problem did not seem to be clearance since his blood levels were stable before suddenly climbing. This had to be a laboratory error or more digoxin administered.

Nancy said that the sentinel event team wanted to know from her how much digoxin he would have to have received to bump his level to 9.61 ng/mL. Bruce and the pharmacist discussed that they could calculate an estimate only by considering the bump as if a single bolus (injection) of drug was administered. Bruce still kept saying that it could be a lab error.

Bruce asked: "What did the ECG show?" The pharmacist stated there was a change in the appearance of the electrocardiogram, but that he suffered a cardiac arrest. She also spoke about a nurse practitioner involved in the sentinel event investigation, Mary Kelly, and stated that the two of them were getting very nervous because there were two people who became unexpectedly hypoglycemic (had low blood sugar) recently while in their intensive care unit.

Bruce offered to have us review the records for them, and Nancy stated she would inform Dr. Cors, the hospital's chief medical officer.

Bruce then stated that he would try to do some calculations, but that his gut told him it was a lab error, or a medication error.

Bruce and I had a lengthy discussion about the situation, and I was extremely skeptical that this could be a laboratory error of that magnitude. It was my feeling that Bruce would continue the discussion with the pharmacist, pharmacist to pharmacist before I intervened.

Bruce called Nancy back that afternoon. He told her that if one calculated a dose based on the premise that the difference was based on a bolus of digoxin administered, then the dose needed to obtain the questioned blood level would have been 2–4 mg of digoxin. With a usual tablet being about 0.25 mg, that translates to ten or more tablets. If administered as an injection it would require 10 mL (about two teaspoons). Most injectable drugs come in a form which require less than 1 mL injections. This would represent a huge medication error if true.

The pharmacist remarked that the patient's heart rate dropped between 6:00 a.m. and 7:00 a.m. from eighty to forty four. She indicated that the question from the sentinel group was "how fast would a heart rate drop from a bolus injection if indeed that was what had transpired?"

Bruce responded, "That would depend on many things, but most importantly was the fact that there is no way that the level could rise that high without him getting more digoxin."

The pharmacist wanted to clarify over what period of time the patient would have to get the 2–4 mg of digoxin. Bruce responded that it is impossible to know. "The calculation depends on a single bolus dose and a level after complete distribution. It takes a while for a medication to become evenly distributed throughout the body." Ruck explained further digoxin tends to concentrate in the heart. Drugs do have predictable patterns of distribution and there is a concept known as "volume of distribution" which explains the relationship between a given dose administered and a blood level measured. One divides the dose administered by the apparent volume of distribution, a figure derived from relating the dose to the blood level of the drug, essentially an indication of the amount medication in the blood versus total body. Unfortunately, it gets very complicated, since when a medication is initially administered by injection into a vein, it does get distributed by the circulation and a level can be measured. It then leaves the circulation and enters tissues and the level may drop quickly. This is known to happen with medications like digoxin. Clinicians generally do not measure digoxin levels until days or even weeks after the medication is started because the relationship doesn't stabilize for that period of time. The clinical situation of this patient made using this conceptual model impossible, so Bruce simply chose the high end in the literature of 6 L/kg to calculate a dose. "To even guess over what time the medication would have to have been administered would be foolish."

The pharmacist then asked Dr. Ruck: "Can you plot a curve and say when the digoxin was administered?"

Bruce, replied: "There may be computer models, but we don't have one, but it is irrelevant. He had to have gotten more digoxin. What makes me real nervous was you telling me of two hypoglycemic patients."

The pharmacist then said, "You probably shouldn't know of the two hypoglycemics." Hypoglycemia means a low blood sugar level. Low blood sugar can be a life-threatening condition if it is very low and if it is not discovered and treated immediately. It can occur from overdoses of insulin, the medicine diabetic patients take to lower their elevated blood sugars, or from an agent which is administered orally and stimulates the body's pancreas to produce and release insulin.

Bruce: "This sounds like it may be a police matter."

The pharmacist ignored Bruce's comment and went back to the discussion of the woman with the mushrooms; her digoxin level on admission was 0.63 and had two "little doses" but on June 16th her digoxin level rose to 9.94 ng/mL at 10 a.m.

Bruce: "What a coincidence of events. This had to be either a huge lab error or more digoxin administered."

The pharmacist stated: "The director of the lab stated they had the levels confirmed in another lab. Now they want me to calculate what dose she would have had to have been given."

Bruce, "Someone had to give her digoxin. If it was given a while before that level was drawn, after it would have had some clearance, her initial level would have been very high and she would have been sick as hell. What else can you tell us about the hypoglycemic patients, did someone measure insulin levels?"

The pharmacist: "Yes, one was really high and an endocrinologist was involved. He looked for an oral hypoglycemic agent." She stated that she did not know the results, nor the result of an assay for "c-peptide." When the body produces insulin in the pancreas, it also produces a protein, c-peptide. If a patient takes an oral hypoglycemic agent, which acts by increasing the pancreas' production of insulin, or if the patient produces more insulin as the result of a tumor or other natural event, there is an increase in both insulin and c-peptide. The pharmaceutical industry produces insulin for administration which is devoid of this c-peptide. Thus, the presence of a high concentration of insulin with low concentrations or even absence of c-peptide strongly suggests that medicinal insulin had to have been administered to a person.

Bruce: "If they had high insulin levels and no c-peptide then someone gave them insulin. Maybe there is a good explanation but if this turns out to be a police matter and the hospital doesn't report it, they will smear the hospital in it." Bruce suggested that we set up a conference call with the hospital's risk manager, Mary Lundt, and their chief medical officer, Dr. Cors, so we could discuss how to proceed.

Pharmacist: "I spoke to the team and offered your (the poison center's) help and Cors said he will call us." She said she would discuss it further with her pharmacy director.

Bruce called the pharmacist back later that afternoon. Bruce: "Is she going to call us?" referring to the hospital's risk manager.

The pharmacist then explained, "I don't know, perhaps she is calling Cors. It was the nurse practitioner and me who got worried with the two hypoglycemic patients."

Bruce: "You are doing the right thing!"

Sometime later the risk manager did call back, and Bruce and I spoke to her. We stated that she needed to call the New Jersey State Department of Health and Senior Services and report a hospital-based outbreak of poisonings. We stated that they also should alert the police. We suggested they get someone from their legal department and their chief medical officer together and we should discuss how to proceed and what role each of us would play. She said that she would get back to us.

On July 9 there was a conference call with the hospital's "team," but no one from their legal affairs group identified themselves as being on the call. The discussion started out again by them asking what dose of digoxin would need to be given to achieve the levels found in the case. Once again, we tried to explain the difficulty in doing this, and the fact that it was irrelevant. Someone had to have administered the medication without authorization. They wanted to get a "handle" so they could possibly look to see if there was drug missing. They confirmed that there were two recent patients who developed unexplained hypoglycemic in their ICU. An endocrinologist stated that there was no explanation except for the administration of exogenous insulin. Bruce and I described the pharmacology of digoxin, stated again that we researched mushrooms concerning digoxin and that we could not find any evidence of mushrooms having any substance which would function and or test as digoxin. We stated that they need to get away from that consideration, that most likely there was someone either making huge mistakes or purposely trying to harm patients. We again suggested they seek legal advice but that we think they need to report to DHSS and the police. Cors asked if we thought that there was anything to be gained by our looking at their records. I responded that we would be happy to, but that this should not delay the reporting of the situation. I pointed out that we did not "want to get caught with our pants down"—that there is a danger that if unreported there could be more deaths and how bad we would all look! I actually told them that these four episodes were sentinel events and they were required to be reported.

On July 10, Chief Medical Officer Cors called. He had the risk manager with him and he spelled out Somerset Medical Center's position that they would begin an investigation into the situation. I tried to explain that this was a serious situation that needed to be reported to the state and the Joint Commission on Accreditation of Healthcare Organizations (JCAHO) immediately. He stated that they were not going to do that until after they investigate, that there are lots of explanations for the lab values. I explained that the mushrooms were not the cause of the increased digoxin levels and the low blood glucose levels. I tried to explain that as a toxicologist and pharmacologist, I felt that there were no explanations to account for the situation. He told me that I was wrong, that the digoxin levels could be the result of drawing blood from the intravenous line. I stated that this would be an incorrect method, and that there was no order for the digoxin to have been given anyway. He then tried to convince me that I didn't understand the pharmacology, that he knew there were logical, scientific explanations. We also discussed the fact that there were four events over about a month's time. I stated that there is no scenario to account for this number of errors except that someone was purposely administering medications, without authorization, to patients. After twenty to thirty contentious minutes of discussion, in frustration, I finally said, "Look, these are sentinel events. They must be reported under state laws and rules of JCAHO." (I did think JCAHO required an immediate report; later JCAHO told me that all that had to be done according to their rules is an investigation started within forty-five days and if anything comes up, then an intervention must then be made.) Dr. Cors kept arguing with me. I then simply stated, "Look, it would look better if Somerset Medical Center reported these events rather than me. I am obligated to report these events through the state, since I am both fiscally responsible, as a program, to the state, and responsible, as a physician, to report any suspected outbreak of nosocomial disease." Dr. Cors then stated, "You do what you have to do, I will do what I have to do. If, after we do a thorough investigation, we feel that we need to call the prosecutor, we will."

Later that day Bruce spoke to the pharmacy director: "Administration has taken over the investigation. They called in attorneys and told us not to speak to any outside agency until after their investigation is done." Bruce asked if the situation had been reported and the administrator said that he didn't know and he was told to refer all calls to risk management. He further stated that "we don't know if we had previous activity. "I feel you guys are forcing their hand inappropriately so for what that's worth. You guys want to remain a viable resource for people so that's, you know, and not be afraid to call." He further stated that "Upper management has come to me and told me that it is an internal investigation…. They brought in legal counsel in on it they are bringing in investigators."

Bruce then came to me and related his conversation with the pharmacy director. I nearly exploded. After I calmed myself down, I called the New Jersey State Epidemiologist and Senior Deputy Commissioner of Health and Senior Services. He was in a meeting and so I left a message. The message I left stated that that I believed there was someone in a hospital in the state trying to kill patients and that I needed to speak to the epidemiologist as soon as possible. Within a reasonably short period of time, he called back and I relayed the story. He asked me why I called him and I stated I did not know who else to call and that since it seemed a nosocomial (hospital) outbreak, I felt he was the correct person to call. He then told me to call Aime Thronton. He was surprised that I had no idea who she was, and he stated she was on the "enforcement side" of the department. He gave me her telephone number. I called and left a voice message for her, also outlining my beliefs that either there was a situation with multiple, serious, life-threatening medical errors, or more likely, that there is someone at Somerset Medical Center trying to kill patients with drugs. She did not call me back that day. After about two hours, when I had not heard from Thronton, I decided to send her an e-mail outlining my fears. The first e-mail came back undeliverable because of a spelling error in her address, but the second time I sent it, she received it. "As the director of the New Jersey Poison Center, I have learned of what appears to be a cluster of four untoward clinical effects over the past two to three weeks at one hospital in New Jersey. In two cases, patients developed toxic levels of digoxin with no documentation of either orders or administration of the drug. In the other two cases there were patients who became severely hypoglycemic and, in at least one, an extremely high level of insulin, which could not have been made by the patient, was found. I spoke to the risk manager of the hospital, the director of pharmacy, the chief operating officer and the chief medical officer and they told me that they were not planning on reporting these incidents to anyone, not the NJDHSS or the police, until they mounted a thorough investigation."

On July 11, I sent an e-mail to the American College of Medical Toxicology's "listserve." The American College of Medical Toxicology is the professional organization of physicians who are board certified in medical toxicology. I explained that there had been a cluster of unusual occurrences at a hospital in New Jersey, two involving high levels of digoxin and two hypoglycemia cases associated with high levels of circulating non-c-peptide insulin. I explained that we had reported the outbreak to the New Jersey Department of Health and Senior Services. I stated that they should be alert to the fact that it is likely they might receive a call regarding the measurement of digoxin, the effect of medical illness on digoxin levels and other similar questions. I was also concerned that the possible perpetrator could leave that hospital undetected and accept a position in another hospital anywhere in the world, and continue his activity attempting to kill patients.

On July 14, Thronton thanked us for sending the report and told us that the department would launch an immediate investigation of the situation at Somerset Medical Center. We asked to be kept in the loop, because we wanted to be sure that all efforts were made to protect the patients. She stated that they would take care of the situation, including reporting it to the police. Several times after that we tried to get copies of the report or any information concerning the circumstances to assuage our feelings that there was an individual trying to kill patients. She told us that when the report was finished she would share it with us.

A few days later we did hear from her and she told us that there were violations found and that the state was deciding on how to handle the situation. We again reminded her of our worries about a poisoner within the hospital.

On July 26 Dr. Cors sent a letter to the state epidemiologist complaining about my actions. He stated that, on our July 10 conference call, "Dr. Marcus was rude, confrontational and adversarial...He did not listen to information presented..." He went on to state that he wanted to alert the state epidemiologist so that "actions can be taken to assure that others seeking the expertise of NJPIES would encounter a valuable resource rather than an adversarial experience."

On August 8, the epidemiologist responded to Cors stating, "it was appropriate for Dr. Marcus to suggest to you that Somerset Medical Center report this case of digoxin toxicity to the NJDHSS" under state statute. He attached a copy of the regulation and a letter from Commissioner Lacy dated May 5, 2003, to all hospitals informing them of their obligation to notify the New Jersey DHSS of reportable events.

On August 7, I presented the cases at the consultant's conference in New York City. It was the consensus of opinion that we were correct in our interpretation that there was a serial murderer involved.

The story then went cold until October 3 of that year. I received a letter from NJDHSS requesting our medical record about the patients which we were consulted on.

On October 27, Detective Daniel Baldwin and Tim Braun from the Somerset County prosecutor's office called the poison center to ask questions about digoxin. He was connected to Bruce.

"Are you talking about the unexplained poisonings at Somerset Medical Center?" asked Bruce.

"What do you know about the cases at Somerset Medical Center?" asked the detectives.

"We called and reported our fears to the NJDHSS that someone was trying to kill patients in Somerset Medical Center's Intensive Care Unit," replied Bruce.

"Can we meet with you and discuss this?" was their immediate reply.

"Sure, come on down!" replied Bruce. Bruce then had me speak to the detectives. I told them that I had developed a loose leaf notebook with the information regarding our experiences with Somerset Medical Center and the cases. They asked if they could come right over, and we stated we would have to consult the University's legal department. We then contacted the university's legal office to get advice on how to proceed. They suggested requesting a formal subpoena. We relayed this information back to the detectives and, soon thereafter, we received a fax copy of a "subpoena duces tecum" from the Somerset County Prosecutor's Office (SCPO). I took the subpoena to our university's legal department to get their approval and suggestion.

Conveniently, that office was located in the same building as our offices. Freda Zackin, an attorney in the legal department of our university was available and I told her the story. She became our ally throughout the following months.

Once we told the detectives that we could and would meet with them, it didn't take long and the two detectives appeared at the office of NJPIES along with a hard, official copy of the "subpoena duces tecum" from the Somerset County Prosecutor's Office (SCPO). Later on, the detectives reported that when they arrived, my statement to them was, "What took you so long?" I am still not sure if I was referring to the several months between the time I made NJDHSS aware of the situation and I assumed that they had learned of it, or if I was referring to their travel time from Somerset to Newark.

The two detectives were amazed at what we told them. We described the entire exchange with the staff at Somerset Medical Center and with New Jersey Department of Health and Senior Services (NJDHSS). We explained that we had been assured by the NJDHSS that if they did not find a logical explanation for the occurrences that they would notify law enforcement. We never did find out exactly how the SCPO became involved. The detectives took a statement from me about the cases.

I was asked by SCPO to review a few charts to see if I could help them understand what had transpired. The first two charts I reviewed had been pulled apart by the detectives so that it was a painful experience trying to reconstruct them to be able to give them my opinions of what transpired.

Over the next several weeks, well into the first week in December, we were in communication with the detectives helping them to understand the medical records we were asked to review. There were multiple cases which appeared to have suffered from sudden events. We reviewed cases for them that had strange outcomes occurring both before our initial report and subsequent to it.

On December 11 the press reported that there was an investigation of a male nurse fired by Somerset Medical Center and that the Somerset County Prosecutor had confirmed that it was investigating.

The story ran in the Newark-based newspaper the *Star-Ledger*:

Officials at the medical center said the nurse in question has a spotty work record during a decade-long career at four hospitals in New Jersey and two in eastern Pennsylvania.

Somerset Medical Center "has conducted an inquiry, as has the New Jersey Department of Health and the New Jersey Poison Control," said Somerset County Prosecutor Wayne Forrest. "We're reviewing their reports. Independently, we're also conducting our own investigation into the deaths that included numerous individual interviews that are still going on."[2]

The next day, Somerset Medical Center released its version of the story: they had asked for references when they hired Mr. Cullen and no one gave them any indication that the nurse had been under any investigation or that there had been any doubt about his qualification to work as a nurse. They stated that it was only after he was "identified as a suspect in the murder of a patient that his troubled background

---

[2] Hepp, R. (2003, December 11) Unexplained deaths at hospital are scrutinized. The Star Ledger, p. 1.

became clear." They never mentioned the call from the poison center calling their attention to the suspicious deaths.

On December 17, Aime Thronton of the NJDHSS sent an email to me thanking me for "spotting the trend" and calling the State's attention to the issue so that an investigation could be pursued.

On December 18, the epidemiologist called NJPIES, spoke to Bruce Ruck stating that he was very upset with the way Somerset Medical Center handled the case and asked for documentation of how, where and when did we state the need to call the police. Bruce sent him our case notes on the incidents.

January 6, 2004, a reporter from the *Star-Ledger* called our offices and told us that Somerset Medical Center sent her a written "time line." In the document Somerset Medical Center claimed that NJPIES was of no help to them. The reporter stated that she would like to ask a series of questions about the situation. I explained that I was told not to speak about the case, but that I would check with the university's attorney for clarification. The attorney working with us, Ms. Zackin, reached out to the Somerset County Prosecutor's Office and was told that, since the case was "actively under investigation," I was not to speak to the press about any of the details. On January 10, I informed the *Ledger* reporter that I was not at liberty to discuss the case with her at this time. She replied: "Ok, I'm not going anywhere... We'll talk someday."

January 14 at 11:46 a.m. the reporter sent me an email to alert me that her newspaper planned to run an article about my "presentation on August 7th to the poison control folks at Bellevue." She wrote: "We talked to three people who were in the audience, two have talked to me or another reporter on the record. We are collaborating, but I will write the story. I understand the legal constraints but we're here, right now. You have declined comment citing the request from the prosecutor's office, Thanks." She further stated that she had a photograph of me presenting at the conference.

January 15 happened to be a snowy day. I carpooled to work with my wife. We had not received our home delivery of the *Star-Ledger* so I did not have access to the newspaper. When I reached the front door of the Bergen Building, I purchased a *Star-Ledger* from a vending machine in the front of the building. There on the front page was a photograph of me from a file the *Star-Ledger* had, not from the presentation, with a big, bold headline which read: "Expert told hospital it had a poisoner, Cullen worked at Somerset Medical Center for three months after it rejected the warning."[3] The phones didn't stopped ringing off of the hook that day. Reporters from all over the globe were calling to get an interview with me. My staff assistant was offered various rewards if she could arrange for an interview. One such offer was from a major television weekly news show offering her dinner in the restaurant of her choice, anywhere she wanted to go, if they could interview me. Of course she was bound to the agreement with the county prosecutor and no such interview was allowed.

---

[3] Campbell CA, Patterson MJ. (2004, January 15). Expert told hospital it had a poisoner. The Star Ledger, p. 1.

That afternoon, January 15, at about 4:30 p.m., I received a telephone call from the New Jersey Commissioner of Health and Senior Services. He related to me how happy he was with the work of NJPIES and stated that my staff is to be congratulated. He then asked questions about ricin (a potential weapon of terrorism), then we chatted about the *Star-Ledger* story. He stated that he received telephone calls from the media asking about the department's activities regarding the situation at Somerset Medical Center. He stated that the *Ledger* called with three specific questions and he related them to me. They wanted to know: (1) when and what did Marcus tell them and in what form and can he release the written documents; (2) if there were no written documents how was the information verbally exchanged; (3) if there was an investigation of the hospital and the investigation showed no explanation for the events, why was nothing done until October? We then chatted about my e-mail to Thronton. He stated that the reason he would not release it, is that it might "embarrass" me because of two spelling errors. I then stated that it might be very embarrassing to the department and that we, NJPIES, myself and UMDNJ have been meeting at length about the situation and consulted with the attorney general and the Somerset County Prosecutor's Office and had written a statement we were using to respond to the press stating that NJPIES followed its regular procedures and reported the situation immediately to the responsible authority (the NJ Department of Health and Senior Services). We further agreed that I was in a unique position as being a material part of the criminal investigation and thus could not discuss the ongoing criminal investigation. I stated that I would have the university's public affairs office send, by fax, a copy of the statement.

Jan 16, 08:22: I sent e-mail to the commissioner with answers to his ricin questions.

Jan 17, 19:40: the commissioner wrote back: "Thank you for the information. Someone from my office will be reaching out to you to schedule a meeting in the near future. Be well."

After Cullen's arraignment a "plea deal" was made that in return for "taking the death penalty off of the table," he would help give "closure" to the families of patients at the various hospitals in which he had worked who died under suspicious circumstances. Cullen agreed to cooperate and admit to murders in addition to those that he was already being charged with. Cullen stated that he would need to be convinced that he had committed the additional murders.

I was asked to review records in which it was unclear if Mr. Cullen had murdered individuals in various hospitals. I was then asked to meet with Mr. Cullen and discuss the cases with him to see if he would be willing to admit to the murders. It was hoped by the SCPO that this would give closure to some families wondering if their loved ones had or had not been victims. On a cold, clear wintry day, I entered a conference room in the court house in Somerset County. There was a television camera and recorder and the two Somerset County Prosecutor's Office detectives, Braun and Baldwin. We discussed what was about to occur and decided upon a strategy to go through the cases one by one and for me to explain what evidence existed in the charts of the dead patients that led me to believe their deaths were other than natural. I was to discuss the cases with Cullen and then he would be asked to admit to their murder at his hands or deny any involvement. After a few minutes of our conversation the door opened and Cullen entered the room. He was dressed in a brown-orange prison jumpsuit, was quiet, and walked to a seat at a table in the conference room across from me. I have been asked on numerous occasions what I felt when I saw him, what did he look like, and was there anything about him that would have drawn any attention to him. I have read many descriptions of other murderers and they all seem to blend into the scenery and do little to attract attention. He fit that description to a "T," he was very non-descript, there was nothing, other than his prison garb, that would have brought any attention to him. When he came into the room and sat at the table, I thought to myself, my goodness, if I walked by him I would not have given him a second glance; I imagined him as the wallflower at a high school dance. He was much shorter and more slender than I had anticipated. He was very quiet and never really initiated any conversation. The detectives explained to him that we would be going through the individual cases and that I would be explaining why I believed that a particular patient had died from unnatural causes and that he would then be given the opportunity to ask questions and then determine if he was willing to admit to the murder. We went through about twenty cases that day. One after the other we discussed the cases and what I believed the putative agent was involved in the deaths. Some were "classic" cases of digoxin overdoses. Digoxin seemed to be one of his preferred agents. Cullen listened closely as I became his instructor in pharmacology and toxicology.

Digoxin is in the class of medications called cardiac glycosides. These medications have their roots in the plant of the genus digitalis, hence the general name given to these is digitalis glycosides as well as being known as cardiac glycosides. Perhaps the most common of such plants is the foxglove, or digitalis purpura. The history of the use of digitalis preparations is fascinating and dates back centuries. It was probably used by early humans for its various effects. Its use as a medicine is attributed to the English physician William Withering who, in 1785 published the landmark book *An Account of the Foxglove, and Some of its Medical Uses With Practical Remarks on Dropsy, and Other Diseases*. Withering was an astute clinician and reported on the beneficial effects of the medication but also warned of the potential toxicities, reporting that about 18% of his patients developed toxicity. The medication became somewhat of the standard of care for many heart problems, from dropsy, heart failure, to arrhythmias, irregular heartbeats. With present understanding of the pathophysiology of cardiac disease, and the problems with toxic effects of the medication, it is not often used anymore. Today its primary use is as a second line agent in treating patients with irregular heartbeats from abnormalities in the atrial beat, the initiation of the normal heart beat from the upper chambers of the heart. Interestingly, because its use cannot be shown to improve mortality and is associated with such a high incidence of toxic side effects, it is unusual for it to be used as the first line treatment for heart failure, the indication made famous by Withering.

The medication possesses a very narrow therapeutic index, or safety window, the difference between its therapeutic and toxic dose. Its mechanism of action makes death by overdose somewhat difficult to prove without tissue levels. Cardiac muscle, like all muscle, exists in an electrical state ready for a nerve impulse to hit its plasma membrane, the covering of the cell. There is an ion pump which pumps potassium into the cell and sodium out of the cell. This is done in such a way that more sodium is pumped out then potassium in. The difference in electric charge is called the membrane potential. The pump is driven by energy obtained from metabolism, adenosine triphosphate, better known as ATP. The pump is named after this energy source and its effect, as the Na/K ATPase pump. Sitting there ready to work is the cardiac muscle. An action potential arrives at the cell membrane and causes the reversal of the pump's action and the rapid movement of sodium into the cell and potassium out. The entering sodium then opens the adjacent calcium channel and is accompanied by the rapid movement of calcium into the cell. The calcium is carried by an intracellular mechanism to the muscle fibers which in the presence of the added calcium then contract. The contraction is then coordinated between muscle cells and the heart itself contracts, expelling blood through its valves through the body. This results in a stronger contraction of the muscles of the heart and slowing of the heartbeat. The cardiac glycosides all have similar effects, they alter the activity of the Na/K ATPase pump and increase the intracellular sodium and calcium and a transiently elevated potassium level in the blood. With normal doses this elevation will not be problematic. The potassium, as well as the medication itself, is eliminated through the kidneys into the urine. In contrast, overdose, as in poisoning, alters the pump in every muscle in the body and produces a significant irregular heart beat and elevated potassium levels of a life threatening potential. In 1977, in a landmark study of patients who suffered from acute poisonings with the medication, Bismuth and her coworkers in Paris demonstrated that toxicity to these medications is accompanied by measureable increases in potassium in the blood. In fact, they reported that a predictor of potential mortality was not the level of actual glycoside found in the blood, but the level of potassium. They demonstrated that none of the victims with potassium levels less than 5.0 meq/L died, 50% of victims with potassium levels between 5.0 and 5.5 meq/L died, 100% of the victims of overdose who had blood levels of potassium of over 5.5 meq/L died. There was little that could be done for those patients at that time. Attempts to lower the potassium, or to keep the heart pumping at its proper rate, did not seem to help. Survival from such poisonings became possible only after an effective antidotal therapy was devised. Smith first reported the successful use of an antibody to the medication in his classic article in the *New England Journal of Medicine* in 1976. This antibody, produced in sheep, was effective almost at any phase of the toxicity but was most effective when administered early. It became commercially available in 1986.

An interesting side effect of the medications in "this class" is the cardiac glycosides are ocular effects, sometimes called "scintillating scotomata." Some refer to this visual disturbance as xanthopsias, flashing colors of light or disturbance of color vision (mostly yellow and green). Some authorities believe that Vincent van Gogh's "Yellow Period" was influenced by his use of digitalis therapy either for his apparent psychosis or in combination with absinthe for its mind altering activity which made the awareness of the environment often startling. The scotomata which are produced is attributed as the effect seen in van Gogh's *The Starry Night*. Van Gogh's digoxin use is supported by multiple self-portraits and portraits of his friends and colleagues which include the presence of examples of the plant, foxglove, from which digoxin is obtained (see, e.g., *Portrait of Dr. Gachet*).

At the end of the session, after Cullen left the room, Braun turned to me and said: "You look strange." I replied that the experience was very peculiar to me. He then asked: "Is this the first time you have met a serial killer?" I sat there speechless for a moment or two then replied, "Are you kidding me? How many people have ever knowingly met a serial killer?"

Although digoxin was frequently Mr. Cullen's preferred poison, he used a variety of medications during his nefarious career. Among the others he utilized were epinephrine (a.k.a., adrenalin), which, in overdose, can so stress the heart that it causes stunning of the heart muscle and causes it to fail producing death. In the 2004 movie *Million Dollar Baby*, which is about a female prize fighter's rise to fame and eventual demise, the death of the main character occurs when epinephrine is injected in a large dose to cause euthanasia. Cullen was also known to add a powerful neuro-muscular blocking agent, succinylcholine, to random bags of intravenous fluids, so that patients receiving the tainted bag would develop paralysis of their muscles and die from inability to breathe.

Sometime after Cullen's trial, after he was incarcerated in state prison, he was sent case files to review in hope that he might shed some light on open cases to again put closure on those cases. His review of one such case included the following statement: "At the time and date of death on Jan 15th according to Dr. Marcus NJ Poison Control and literature any acute large dose of digoxin would cause drastic increase in K+ (potassium) level. So while digoxin and my involvement is ruled out by normal K levels in hospital chart."

Were there missed opportunities to have stopped the killings? Of course there were. One such was a death in another hospital in July 1996. Review of the hospital record from that incident revealed the following note in the summary of the chart after the death of an eighty-year-old man: "Of interest and unexplained is a rising Dig level given the fact that his initial dig level was 3 and rose to 10. Unfortunately, this brought up the question of a possibility of Dig toxicity but that does not explain why it continued to rise."

There is a long history of healthcare workers who murdered patients. What leads an individual to perform these horrendous acts is unknown.

Postscript

The attempt by Somerset Medical Center to deflect blame onto the institutions who had Cullen as an employee and did not warn subsequent institutions of his poor performance led to the legislature examining the events leading up to Cullen's arrest. The New Jersey legislature passed legislation protecting nursing homes and hospitals from legal action when reporting disciplinary actions taken against employees. Further, it required workers to report co-workers whose actions are questionable.

There is still no law which stipulates mandatory reporting of multiple deaths in a hospital. Unless they are of infectious origin, drug or chemical exposures resulting in death are not reportable to the NJDHSS, actually now called the New Jersey department of Health (NJDoH).

Retelling the Story

In the spring of 2012, I received a telephone call from an investigative reporter, Charles Graeber. He said that he was working on a book about Cullen and asked to meet with me. He sent samples of his previous work, so that I could examine them and determine that he was a legitimate author. We met several times, sharing information that I had accumulated over the course of time after the initial confrontation with the hospital. His book, *The Good Nurse*, was published in April 2013. He sent me a signed copy with the inscription "A little sunshine is the best medicine sometimes. Here's to lifting rocks and peering underneath."

I could never understand why the Department of Health failed to act after I called and reported my fears that there was someone murdering patients at Somerset Medical Center. In a conversation that I had with the state epidemiologist at that time of the Cullen incident, the epidemiologist stated that we would sit and discuss the situation "sometime" in the future and see what went right and wrong and why his department did not act. He subsequently left the department of health to work in the pharmaceutical industry and never responded to any of my invitations to sit and speak about the events. In Graeber's book, in the notes at the end of the book, there are some compelling, if not damning statements. Graeber opined that "the process of reporting, investigating, and ultimately acting upon the incidents at Somerset Medical Center in a timely manner had been stalled or sidetracked at several junctures, both within Somerset Medical Center and at the highest level of the DoH itself." Graeber further stated: "The sitting Commissioner of Health and Senior Services at the time was Cliff Lacey. According to e-mails from the senior assistant commissioner, Marilyn Dahl, the incidents at Somerset Medical Center had been discussed with Commissioner Lacey following the reporting of both Steven Marcus and then Somerset Medical Center administrators. 'Based on his experience with the drugs in question, and as the senior medical officer in a large hospital, the commissioner thought that it was extremely premature to start suspecting foul play. I had, at that time, raised the issue of a referral to the AG, and the commissioner declined.' Dahl wrote, "He was able to hypothesize several likely scenarios not involving foul play that could have resulted in the outcomes reported." Graeber went on in the notes to quote Dahl as saying that she had met with several members of the DoHSS staff and: "We all agreed that there may be sufficient reason to suspect foul play. The disturbing part of the picture is that Somerset had made us aware of the three previous occurrences, yet chose to wait an entire month before reporting the third. We believe that this was irresponsible at best, and would like permission to seek counsel's opinion from OLRA (the DOH office of Legal and Regulatory Affairs] for referral to the AG's (Attorney General's] office."

The release of the book revived interest in Cullen. The television news magazine show *60 Minutes* received permission for an interview with Cullen. The show was aired and included interviews with Graeber, Cullen, the nurse who helped collect evidence and convince Cullen to cooperate with the prosecutor, and me. The interviewer spent a great deal of time going over how I became involved and when and why I suspected foul play. He asked if I was upset by the delay and the fact that several individuals died between my alerting the hospital and the DoHSS of my suspicions and I "teared up." All of my friends, family, and colleagues knew of the *60 Minutes* interview and sat glued to their television sets while the interviewer discussed the fact that a "government bureaucrat," me, had been responsible for setting the wheels in motion which eventually resulted in Cullen's arrest. No one who knows me could ever imagine me being called a bureaucrat!

Suggested Reading

Bismuth C, Gaultier M, Conso F, Efthymiou L. Hyperkalemia in acute digitalis poisoning: prognostic significance and therapeutic implications. Clin Toxicol. 1973;6(2):153–62.
Graeber C. The good nurse. New York: Hachette Book Group; 2013.
Smith TW, Butler VP, Haber E, et al. Treatment of life-threatening digitalis intoxication with digoxin-specific fab antibody fragments. N Engl J Med. 1982;307(22):1357–62.
Yang EH, Shah S, Criley JM. Digitalis toxicity: a fading but crucial complication to recognize. Am J Med. 2012;124:337–43.

Chapter 6
Screams from a Glass Coffin

Thanksgiving Day at New Jersey Poison Information and Education System progressed as it had for many years before. Calls from frightened people when they realized they forgot to remove the bag of organs from inside the turkey before baking it. Others asked what temperature and for how long to cook the turkey. All in all things were pretty quiet. The next day was filled with the usual assortment of poison center calls punctuated by those people who thought they may have developed food poisoning from the meal. Although it is never really boring at the poison hotline, the work is often tedious. Things were about to change a bit for the medical director and staff of the poison center.

Rolando Diaz, the poison information specialist on duty, received a telephone call from Dr. Montalban, an emergency medicine physician, at eleven-fifteen at night the day after Thanksgiving. He was calling to discuss the care of a young female patient in his emergency department who was transported by ambulance to the hospital. The story he related was that his patient was given a "Botox" treatment to remove wrinkles by her friend, who was allegedly a physician, in Florida two days prior to this incident. According to the story he relayed, her friend also had the treatment. The friend told the Emergency Department physician that the preparation was "incorrectly diluted" and that she received 800 units (the usual vial only contains 100 units so this history was discounted). On the day of the Emergency Department visit, the patient developed difficulty breathing and they called for an ambulance. In transit she developed what was described as "respiratory distress" and was administered epinephrine, also known as adrenalin, a medication used to treat serious allergic reactions and which helps to promote dilatation of the airway. In the Emergency Department she was having noisy, obstructive-sounding respirations. To treat this, an airway tube was inserted into her trachea (breathing pipe), and she was sedated with the drug (Diprivan® propofol) and placed on a mechanical ventilator. At the time of the call to the poison center she was sedated, her vital signs showed a slightly low blood pressure of 109/75, and a slightly elevated heart rate of 102.

Rolando called me, the on-call toxicologist, and I was "conferenced" into a conversation with Dr. Montalban. There was marked confusion about what actually

© Springer International Publishing AG 2017
S.M. Marcus, *Medical Toxicology: Antidotes and Anecdotes*,
DOI 10.1007/978-3-319-51029-3_6

had transpired. Although I had heard of cases in which there were some untoward events from Botox, there had been none that I knew of with this degree of severity. Additionally, I had never heard of diluting Botox, the brand name preparation marketed for cosmetic use by the pharmaceutical company Allergan. I asked Dr. Montalban to describe exactly what he heard and saw which led him to intubate the patient. Dr. Montalban demonstrated the sound he heard which sounded like respiratory obstruction to me. Interestingly, the EMS crew obviously thought the same, that she had constriction of her bronchial tree, and they treated her with epinephrine en route as if she were having a severe asthma attack. This is not what I would have expected if "Botox" had been the causal agent, since it causes muscle paralysis and hence the patient's respirations would become depressed, not stimulated, and her airway would have become relaxed not constricted.

Clostridium botulinum, the bacteria that produces this toxin, has been known to cause muscle paralysis for over a hundred years. In 1897 the physician Justinus Kerner first described the bacterium associated with poorly prepared meats, calling it botulinum or "sausage poison." There are eight serologically distinct toxins produced by the bacteria, named A through H. Botox is the proprietary name for a preparation of botulinum toxin type A. The botulinum toxin has the potential to cause paralysis by interfering with nerve conduction across the neuro-muscular junction. When a nerve impulse moves along a motor nerve, those nerves which communicate to muscles to contract, the nerve impulse, causes the movement of an intra-cellular vesicle containing acetylcholine, a neurotransmitter since it transmits the neural impulse, to the cell membrane. Once this vesicle attaches to the cell membrane, the vesicle opens into the space between the nerve ending and the muscle, releases the acetylcholine and the muscle contracts. Botulinum toxin consists of a two chain polypeptide, a heavy and a light chain. The heavy chain appears responsible for the toxin adhering to the exterior of the nerve ending by binding to proteins on the surface of the axon terminal, the end of the nerve. The light chain is cleaved off of the heavy chain and is then able to move internally by a process called endocytosis, the formation of a cyst-like structure containing the light chain, or the active part of the toxin. Once inside the cytoplasm of the nerve cell, the toxin is released from the endocyst. This toxin then alters the mechanism which is responsible for the movement of the acetylcholine vesicle, rendering it unable to bind to the cell membrane. The toxin changes the shape and denatures the protein responsible for fusing the acetylcholine-containing vesicle to the end of the axonal terminal, a sort of docking station. Failure to "dock" prevents the release of acetylcholine, the neurotransmitter, and thus prevents further movement of the nerve impulse and prevents muscle contraction. This causes flaccid, sagging, paralysis of the affected muscle. The toxin can affect virtually every muscle in the body which requires a nerve impulse to contract, thus total paralysis is what will be seen clinically.

There are approximately 145 cases of botulism reported to the United States Centers for Disease Control and Prevention (CDC) each year.[1] There are three major forms of clinical botulism. Adult, dietary botulism, representing approximately

---

[1] Botulism, General Information, National Center for Emerging and Zoonotic Infectious Diseases, CDC http://www.cdc.gov/nczved/divisions/dfbmd/diseases/botulism/ accessed 7 May 2016.

15% of the reported cases, occurs when food is contaminated with the spore form of botulinum bacteria. Under correct temperature and oxygen concentrations (the spore prefers little or no oxygen and a warm environment), the spores contaminating the food will germinate into a "vegetative form," that is the form that produces the toxin. This often occurs when individuals incorrectly prepare fish, can vegetables, or let foods ferment incorrectly. Ingesting the spores themselves in adults rarely causes any problem, since the stomach acid tends to prevent the germination of the spores. The ingestion of food contaminated with toxin results, after a period in which the toxin is distributed throughout the body, in the patient developing muscle weakness. Usually such weakness starts proximally, in the nerves that control eye movement, producing double vision. There is often first a feeling of a sore throat followed by difficulty swallowing and progressive movement of paralysis into the rest of the body. There is antitoxin available for treatment, but to be effective it must be administered very early in the course of the illness. Unfortunately, since the disease is so rare, the diagnosis is usually delayed or not made until additional individuals who consumed the same food present for care.

There is an infant form of botulism, which represents approximately 65% of all reported cases of botulism, in which an infant ingests the spores themselves. Spores are somewhat ubiquitous in nature, often found in dirt and soil. The association between botulinum spores and honey is well known. Infants' stomach juices are inadequate in acidity to prevent the germination of the bacterium. If a certain quantity of spores is ingested, they will germinate and produce an infection within the intestines and the vegetative form will reproduce within the intestines and will produce the toxin. The absorption of toxin results in paralysis similar to that in adults. The children often present with decreased muscle tone, difficulty sucking a nipple or breast, and constipation. As with the adult dietary form, antidotal therapy is useful for infants. There is a specific antidote intended for the infant form which is particularly effective. The antitoxin used for infant form (BabyBIG©) is made by the California Department of Health and is based on human blood samples, while that intended for adults is of equine (horse) origin. If the diagnosis of infant botulism is made early the apparent reversal of the paralysis by BabyBIG© can be dramatic. Unfortunately, once the toxin has moved inside the nerve cell and disrupts the docking station, the toxin's action cannot be reversed. Often the diagnosis of botulism is delayed beyond the point in which antitoxin therapy is of any use.

There is a third form of botulism, which is similar to that of infant botulism since it is really an infection, but it is caused by skin wounds becoming contaminated with spores. This is often the result of "skin popping" of illicit drugs, injecting dirty illicit drugs into the skin to get high. The paralysis is similar to that in the other forms, but since the infection can last a while, the paralysis may be prolonged.

The history of the use of botulinum toxin clinically is very interesting. An ophthalmologist, Alan Scott, became interested in the therapeutic use of botulinum toxin in treating the condition blepharospasm, an extremely debilitating frequent spasmodic contraction of the muscles in the eyelids. He worked with a "micromanufacturer" who extracted minute concentrations of the toxin and injected it into his patients with amazing relief. The indication for such treatment was expanded to include cases of strabismus, crossed eye, in which one set of eye muscles was weakened by injection to enable the eyes to become coordinated. The micromanufacturer was unable to keep up with the demand and the legal obstacles of producing the drug and in 1989 the manufacturer Allergan introduced a United States Food and Drug Administration (FDA) approved preparation of botulinum toxin type A, which they called "Botox." The use of Botox rapidly spread when in 2002, the FDA agreed to expand its indications to include removal of frown marks and wrinkles.

Dr. Montalban asked if he should remove the artificial airway. "No way," I replied, "let us just leave well enough alone at this point while we sort out what actually happened." When I asked how the friend was, I was told that he was fine and was going to be sent home.

At 10 a.m. the following morning, Richard Casas, the information specialist on duty at the New Jersey Poison Center, received a call from Lewis Nelson, a toxicologist at the New York City Poison Center (NYCPCC), just across the river from the New Jersey Poison Control Center in Newark, New Jersey. The NYCPCC had received a call from the same hospital about a male patient with "botulism" who was admitted to the hospital. This poison center received information that the male patient, a physician, had injected himself with Botox and claimed that the Botox had not been properly diluted. The NYCPCC attempted to get botulinum antitoxin from the United States Centers for Disease Control for the patient and was told that the New Jersey Health Department of Health and Senior Services (NJDHSS) had to make the formal request and so Nelson called NJPIES to have me become involved and to call the NJDHSS. Casas called me and I was able to speak to Nelson. He did not know about the female patient. It became clear that there were two patients in the same hospital with a clinical condition in which there was consideration of the diagnosis of botulism from a rather unusual possible source.

I called the hospital and spoke to the consulting neurologist, Dr. Ivan Klein (a pseudonym). The story of the presentation and physical examination seemed bizarre. Since it was a holiday weekend, I was tied up with visiting family and could not break away immediately but offered to go to the hospital and see the patient. They were concerned about the patient and asked that I see her and give them my opinion.

My daughter, Leigh, then a medical student at the Medical College of Virginia, was home for the holiday. I had to drive her to Newark Airport for a flight back to Richmond, Virginia, and then I would go to the hospital and see the patient. I spoke to Marsha Train (a pseudonym), a physician who worked for the United States Centers for Disease Control and Prevention (CDC). She was assigned as a CDC Epidemic Intelligence Officer (EIS) to the New Jersey Department of Health and Senior Services. I suggested that she meet me at the hospital and we would examine and assess the patients together. Arriving at the hospital, I found the EIS officer already at the bedside. Considering the preliminary diagnosis, we observed some unexpected findings in both of the New Jersey index patients in the intensive care unit. The female patient was on ventilator support but had some reflex activity in her arms and could, ever so slightly, move her great toes in response to questioning. Her pupils were 6–8 mm in diameter, the widest is 10 mm and is what I expected to see if she was paralyzed from botulism since it paralyzes all muscles of the body, with no response to light. Her "doll's eye response" also known as the vestibular-ocular reflex (VOR), was abnormal. In this reflex, the examiner moving the patient's head rapidly in one direction should produce eye movement in the direction opposite to head movement, preserving the image on the center of the visual field. For example, when the head moves to the right, the eyes move to the left, and vice versa. Since slight head movement is present all the time, this reflex action is very important for stabilizing vision. Patients whose VOR is impaired find it difficult to read, because they cannot stabilize their eyes. The VOR does not depend on visual input and works even in total darkness or when the eyes are closed. She also had bilaterally absent cold caloric tests. This is another test used to assess damage to the ear or the brainstem. When cold or warm water is put into the external ear canal, the eyes move via reflex action, unless there is either ear or brain damage. In botulism, the muscles which move the eyes in the orbits are paralyzed and thus the eyes do not move even with this stimulation. Her muscle strength was non-existent, and her muscles felt like balloons filled with water, without any palpable muscle mass. She was having what appeared to be rather violent spasms, which looked like opisthoto-nus, or excessive arching of her back muscles, and she had tight Achilles tendons bilaterally. In addition, it was near impossible to open her jaw even minimally, and the staff had to use a wedge to prevent her from biting through the breathing tube which had been inserted through her mouth and into her airway. The male patient, in contrast, was in significantly less distress, and was sitting up in bed watching television.

While we were in the intensive care unit, a telephone call was received from CDC to find out how the patients were doing. The CDC person was calling about two patients in their fifties. This puzzled me and caused me to interrupt the caller, "wait a minute, are you discussing two patients in New Jersey?" The CDC person then said, "No, in Florida." I then remarked, "Are you saying that you know of two patients, a male and a female, in their fifties, in Florida, who have what may be clini-cal botulism from injections of Botox?"[2] The caller then confirmed this fact. It appeared that there was an outbreak of an apparent disease, of a neurological nature, associated with injection of "Botox" in Florida resulting in two patients being hos-pitalized in Florida and two in New Jersey.

Shortly after the telephone call, a gentleman, Dr. Emanuel Tolia (a pseudonym), stating that he was a partner of the male patient, arrived to see him and speak about the problem. As it turned out, Dr. Tolia was the owner of the facility in Fort Lauderdale, Florida, in which both of the New Jersey patients worked. The female was employed as a massage therapist and the male was an unlicensed physician. Dr. Tolia's son, allegedly a medical student, had somehow been involved with a dilution of "Botox." Dr. Tolia said that he was really not sure who gave the injections, and wondered if another unlicensed physician working at the spa may have actually administered the Botox to the patients. He stated that the male patient in Florida was a consultant to his practice, a chiropractor who gave lectures on increasing the prof-

[2]This discussion is a recreation of the conversation based on contemporaneous notes made by me and later entered into the electronic medical record kept at the poison center.

itability of the office. Dr. Tolia spoke about how they hoped to help with the possessions of the two patients which were at the home of our male patient's mother in New Jersey. According to Dr. Tolia, when the Florida couple first became ill, his son went to their home and administered an infusion of Myers Cocktail to them.

I called the medical toxicologist that I knew at the poison center located in Florida. The Florida center did not have a great deal of information and they did not have anyone who actually saw the patients. I provided him with the information we had obtained and gave him the benefit of my physical examination.

At some time during the first few days of the female's hospitalization, her sister told the treating staff that when the sisters were very young, growing up in rural Alabama, they often shared the same bed. So that their parents didn't find out that they were awake, they would silently spell out words using body movements and answering questions as yes or no. Her sister demonstrated how to communicate with our patient using her ability to move her great toe as meaning yes. To spell out what she wanted to tell us we would then ask her if she wanted to "talk to us." If she motioned yes, we would then start spelling words, A to L, yes or no, then M to Z painstakingly narrowing down each letter in a word and each word in a phrase which she was able to communicate to us. Amazingly, she was able to keep track well enough of what she was spelling to enable us to have "complete conversations" with her. The efforts were tedious, but allowed us to learn about clinical effects she was experiencing and what her desires and needs were, such as managing her pain syndrome.

The investigation of the Florida cases was paralleling what we were doing in New Jersey. The Florida patients, husband and wife, became ill on Thanksgiving Day. They thought that they were coming down with "the flu." They played golf that day. The following day they developed difficulty swallowing, muscle weakness, and abnormal lung function tests and were admitted to the hospital. The Florida Epidemic Intelligence Service Officer interviewed the Florida patients' son and learned that he had been in the room during the time his parents were injected. He reported that his mother received four or five injections while he couldn't remember how many his father received. He stated that late the night before Thanksgiving his parents complained of 'feeling rummy," with dry mouth, blurred vision, and generalized weakness. He said that after Dr. Tolia administered Myers' Cocktails to his parents, they became immobile. The EIS officer reported that he examined the patients and found paralysis of cranial nerves but intact peripheral musculature.

The Florida Department of Health became involved in an investigation of the spa owned by Dr. Tolia and in which the two New Jersey patients worked. The spa had purchased "Botox," but the manufacturer only had records showing two vials ever being shipped there. At that time, Botox was ordered directly from and was shipped by the manufacturer. This raised the issue of what was truly given to the patients in Florida.

The fifth day of her illness, the New Jersey female patient was transferred to the New Jersey hospital in which I practiced. She was no longer having muscle spasms and was completely flaccid. She did have some volitional movement of her toes and her deep tendon reflexes were present, although decreased, in her upper extremities. She had absent bowel sounds and was "complaining" of being hungry.

On day seven, her sister visited the hospital and complained that the family could not gain access to her personal effect, that is her clothing, jewelry, purse and her identification, at the friend's house. I called the local police to ask them to look into the situation, the possibility that there might be some evidence of a crime at the home. The police took the information and said they would call me back. When I had not heard anything for several days, I called the Federal Bureau of Investigation. I mistakenly believed at that time that, since there were cases across state lines, two in Florida and two in New Jersey, this should be a federal investigation. The agent on call told me that this would not be a federal case, but that I should call the New Jersey State Police. When I called the State Police, I was told that this would be a county jurisdiction, not state. When I then called the County Prosecutor's office, I was told that since there was no death, the investigation would have to be initiated by the local police and only if they then requested county involvement or if there was a death, would the county become involved. I then called the local police again and was told that the desk sergeant would let the captain know. I was later informed that the police, upon visiting the home, could not locate the personal belongings of the patient.

The neurology service at my hospital did electromyographic (EMG) and nerve conduction studies. The results showed total denervation of all muscles tested; there was no sign that any nerve impulses were getting to the muscle, hence the muscle paralysis. There is normally some nervous stimulation of the muscles which support the skeleton. In botulism, all of the nerve endings between the nerves and the muscles, the so called neuromuscular junction, are paralyzed. The EMG confirmed that finding in our patient. The neurologist then increased the intensity of the electrical shock he imparted onto the nerves to determine if he could force any conduction into her muscles. This showed no change in amplitude with repeated high intensity stimulation. The patient later remarked that this was the most painful experience of her life, and said she was screaming internally and no one could hear her, as if she were "screaming from a glass coffin."

The male patient considered a transfer to my hospital as well, and sent his brother and friend to see the facility. The friend, a chiropractor, was an "expert" in alternative medicine, including mesotherapy, and had suggestions for therapies to be used. The decision was made not to transfer. He stayed at the original hospital.

Meanwhile the investigation about the "Botox" involved in the outbreak was continuing. The FDA became the lead agency in the investigation. They organized a "raid" on the spa to obtain records and any possible evidence for what transpired. Toxicologists from the Florida Poison Center accompanied the FDA officers in the raid. They found vials of botulinum neurotoxin Type A, manufactured by Toxin Research International, Inc., located in Tucson, Arizona. The vials were labeled "FOR RESEARCH PURPOSES ONLY" and also "NOT FOR HUMAN USE." Interestingly enough, although there is no recognized way to provide a dose in weight terms, the standard being "mouse units" (even the branded Botox lists the preparation as 100 units in a vial, not a certain weight of toxin), this vial stated that it contained 500 units and also stated that this was five nanograms, or five billionth of a gram which is about one five hundredth of a pound. The FDA looked into the background of this Toxin Research International. They had been producing this product for some time. Additionally, they had sponsored seminars for physicians during which they stated that the preparation is produced under the same guidelines as the branded product and their staff suggested that it could be used interchangeably. They shipped many vials of this preparation to physicians throughout the United States. Tracking back their supplier—that is, who actually provided the raw botulinum toxin that Toxin Research International produced—we found that a California based company, List Biological Laboratories, produced a Botulinum Neurotoxin Type A from clostridium botulinum, which they sold in vials of 100 µg of powder. If the weight and units could in fact be calculated, then the brand name Botox vials would contain an index quantity of 100 units, the Toxin Research International five units, but the List preparation in excess of ten million units! At that time, all three preparations were being sold for about 500 dollars each. It is easy mathematics to see the cost savings and increased profit one could achieve by simply diluting the higher concentration to produce a "counterfeit Botox." Unfortunately, it would take gallons of diluent to bring the ten million units down to a usable concentration similar to the brand name, and the risk for miscalculation and potential harm extremely great. FDA agents in Tucson were able to obtain records for the vials shipped from that company. There were then nationwide attempts to find the vials in the possession of physicians and to confiscate them, before more victims appeared.

On the tenth day of hospitalization my patient had regained enough muscle strength that she was able to move her upper arms, primarily the brachio-radialis muscle group. In addition she demonstrated some extra-ocular movement but had a persistent nerve paralysis of her facial muscles. There was a suggestion of an abdominal reflex; when I stimulated the skin of her abdomen, there was an ever so slight movement of the abdominal musculature. I also was able to hear scattered bowel sounds, an optimistic sign that her intestines might soon be capable of her being fed.

The patient's progress in the intensive care unit was complicated by repeated aspiration pneumonia (fluid from her stomach and saliva from her mouth would trickle into her airway around the tube placed there for her breathing) and caused infection in her lungs. Every time we tried to raise her head up from the supine position, she developed hypotension (low blood pressure) and light headedness to the extent that her head had to be lowered. She complained of being uncomfortable in the bed: "This bed sucks." She complained of feeling as if she was on a "roller coaster" when she received pain medication, and requested that such medication be kept to a minimum, but she did complain of severe headaches. She began on feedings through a tube inserted through her nose and into her stomach. Unfortunately, since her stomach and intestines were paralyzed, the "food" pooled up in her stomach and never progressed into her intestines. There was a large amount of residual fluid in her stomach which would back up and end up in her lungs.

On the seventeenth day of hospitalization, she underwent elective tracheostomy, the placement of a hole into her trachea (windpipe) to allow a device, a tracheostomy tube, to be placed into the hole that could be attached to a mechanical ventilator. This would allow the tube placed into her windpipe to be removed and, we hoped, would make her a little more comfortable. A plastic feeding tube was placed through the skin of her abdomen into her stomach to enable the removal of the tube through her nose and allow us to feed her directly into her stomach or intestines. This would allow, we hoped, for better "comfort care."

On hospital day twenty she was able to move her hips slightly and move her legs apart. She complained of headache and ear blockage. Physical examination revealed a fluid level in her left middle ear. Since she was still demonstrating some degree of autonomic instability (exaggerated response to stress), we were reluctant to use local vasoconstrictors to help with her eustachian tube and started her on intranasal steroids instead. We hoped this would decrease swelling of the surroundings of the eustachian tubes and allow the eustachian tubes to function correctly. She was started on lorazepam (Ativan) for anxiety and ketorolac (an injectable nonsteroidal analgesic similar to such drugs as ibuprofen or Advil) for pain.

On the twenty-first hospital day she stated her headache was worse and we tried to begin her on morphine, but she did not tolerate it so we switched to a fentanyl patch. She did not like the feeling she got from the fentanyl and it was discontinued after a day. After many attempts at managing her pain, she felt the most relief with the least side effects with (Dilaudid hydromorphone hydrochloride), an older medication in a similar class to morphine. Although we warned her not to wait until the pain was severe before asking for it, the fact that she didn't like to feel spacey and the difficulty she had in communicating her needs with the staff produced an inefficient mechanism to control her pain.

Once "trached," and apparently able to better tolerate being moved and cared for by regular nursing staff, she was moved to a subacute care unit. "F-yellow" was such a unit with a large percentage of patients "graduates" of the intensive care unit. These patients, primarily ventilator-dependent patients, are housed in this unit so that they can be watched closely but not at the intensity afforded patients in the ICU. The patient was placed in a private room not far from the nursing station. Generally, she was assigned to a nurse who had few other patients to take care of. Unfortunately, most nursing staff are used to patients that appear the same as this young woman, who arrive in that state because of either something they did to themselves and or are likely to not achieve a normal life after their hospitalization. Often termed "gomers," or "gorks," derogatory slang terms used derived from the saying get out of my emergency room, or god only really knows. Such patients are not exactly looked upon as desired ones to care for.

Knowing that this was often the case, we took special precautions to explain to the staff that this young woman was completely aware of what was happening to her, was probably extremely anxious and frightened. We left signs all around the room and on her bed, and even wrote them on her body if she had to go off of the nursing unit for a test, writing the words "I am awake, I know exactly what is happening to me, I feel pain, please be careful with me." We had to explain that she did have normal sleep and awake cycles and had to be treated with the understanding that although she looked to be in coma at all times, she was not. We had to suggest that people speak to her, keep her informed about what was going on around her, that they should not simply assume that she was in coma and couldn't feel pain, etc.

Luckily for her, she developed a small following of "angels." She was adopted by members of a voluntary church organization that provided volunteers to sit and speak to her. One of the physical therapists, Julie, became her real life line. This therapist made it a point to get the patient out of the bed and into a chair. The dental school provided students to help insure good dental hygiene.

Despite Julie's efforts and those of her church guardian angels, the patient's spirits were very low, particularly during Christmas time. Her nutrition support was not working, liquid feedings put into her stomach through her "peg tube" stayed in her stomach because of lack of gastrointestinal motility. If not removed by suctioning, the feeding simply backed up into her esophagus and mouth and had to be suctioned from there lest she aspirate it down her windpipe and into her lungs. She developed a bright red rash which we were able to pin down to a reaction to the skin cream being rubbed on her body to avoid bed sores. She communicated to us that she knew that she had an allergy to some of the skin products and told us which specific one to get for her. We were fortunate in that one of our poison information specialists was taking a course in therapeutic massage and was able to obtain the very lotion that our patient requested.

Two days after Christmas, the patient "told me" that she felt as if she "didn't exist." I pleaded with the nurses to respect the fact that the patient was awake although appeared not to be, and to please go into her room and speak to her, even if they felt silly. I also realized that she really had no way to see anything in the room and that the only functional senses were touch, hearing, and smell. When I realized that, I also realized that hospital rooms have peculiar odors. I went across the street and purchased plug in room deodorizers of different aromas to put into her room. Her angels brought in magazines to read to her and set up regular visits.

By the day of New Year's Eve, she started to rally a bit. She was starting to try to mouth words. This was still not as effective as the way she was spelling words with movements. I wasn't totally sure, but it seemed as if she tried to reach out for my hand. She continued to complain of severe headaches, and was still refusing the medication for it. Her peg tube was not giving her any effective nutrition.

On January 6 she was able to produce what I will call a smile. Her eyes were now functioning, and she could raise her hand off of the bed.

By January 13, she was able to tolerate being out of bed in a chair for one hour before becoming exhausted. A special bed was found that provided preventive movements which would help prevent ulcer formation as well as percussion to help loosen secretions in her lungs. Unfortunately, the mechanisms built into the bed made sounds as if there was a machine gun going off in her room. The pain management team was trying to help us with a variety of medications and physical means to minimize her discomfort. Her peg tube was still ineffective at providing her with any nutrition. We considered the fact that she was receiving opioids for pain management and that perhaps this was interfering with her gastrointestinal tract movements. There are opioids receptors in the gastrointestinal tract. When they are stimulated, the intestines stop contracting. We put naloxone, a medication which reverses the effects of opioids into her stomach through the peg tube. Since the medication is not absorbed through the gastrointestinal tract, it was our hope that it would reverse the local effects of the opioids on the receptors in the gastrointestinal tract without blocking the pain relief. We also added medications to her treatment that usually help promote the movement of the gastrointestines, so called pro-kinetic agents. We were "rewarded" by being able to hear the sounds of movement when we listened to her abdomen with a stethoscope. She even seemed to pass some gas. We optimistically increased the volume of fluid feeding through the peg tube. Alas, however, the stomach still would not empty. We were further disappointed when she was turned down by the rehabilitation institute because she was still on a ventilator and needed total parenteral feedings. They said they would be able to take her with only one of those confounding problems, but not both.

The gastroenterology group attempted to pass a tube through the stomach and into the jejunum, far enough into the intestine that perhaps she might be able to tolerate enteral feeding. They were unsuccessful at accomplishing this at the bedside.

On February 2, the respiratory therapist deflated the cuff on her tracheostomy tube, took her off of the ventilator and she was able to briefly speak. Unfortunately she became short of breath when off of the ventilator and had to be hooked back up. Despite the little setback, her spirits were flying high. She began to see the "light at the end of the tunnel."

On February 9, an X-ray revealed that the peg tube, pushed further by the gastro-enterology group, was now coiled within her stomach. They took her to the operating room where, under anesthesia, they attempted to place the tube into her jejunum and anchor it into place with a suture, a standard operating procedure. The gastro-enterologist remarked that with most individuals, it is easy to simply use a suture to tie the end of the tube in place, because you can use the muscles of the jejunum to grab the needle as you suture. In her situation, the muscles did not respond, because they were still paralyzed from the botulinum toxin.

Walking into her room the afternoon of February 19 was an astonishing experience, given where "she had been." She was moving around in her bed. She was still having trouble swallowing even her own minimal oral secretions, but she could reach out for the suction tubing and was able to suction out her own mouth. She was beginning to say that her pain had decreased and now she was complaining about the sounds of the monitors, alarms, etc. She also began refusing to use the bed's built in percussion.

On March 7 she was able to stand and hold onto a walker. She now tolerated peg feedings and did not require total parenteral nutrition. On March 9, her 105th hospital day, she was accepted into the rehabilitation center.

She was to remain on a ventilator intermittently at the rehabilitation center, able to breathe on her own while awake but requiring the ventilator at night for several weeks. Eventually she tolerated removal of the ventilator and the tracheostomy tube was removed. She was discharged from the rehabilitation center to live with her father in her home state of Alabama.

A year after her discharge from care in New Jersey, she returned to pay a visit and to thank those who were instrumental in saving her life. Her greatest desire during her hospitalization was to leave the hospital and go to the Cheesecake Factory and buy everyone cheesecake. One of her first stops upon returning to New Jersey was a stop for lunch at the Cheesecake Factory! During the visit she told me that she was writing a book and that the title was originally going to be "Screams from a Glass Coffin" but she changed it to simply "From a Glass Coffin." She gave me the "go ahead" to use the title "Screams from a Glass Coffin." From the mouth of the victim came the best title.

Postscript

The FDA's Office of Criminal Investigation (OCI) launched an investigation into the situation. In total there were over 200 investigations of physicians throughout the United States. It is estimated that over a thousand individuals were injected with the preparation sold by Toxin Research International, labeled "For Research Only, Not for Human Use. The OCI investigation eventually led to 31 arrests and 29 convictions of individuals who purposely injected unlicensed botulinum toxin into individuals without the knowledge that they were receiving such an unlicensed product. Charges ranged from the use of an unlicensed preparation to conspiracy, mail fraud and misbranding of a drug to making false statements, etc. Toxin Research International and its owners, and the male patient in this outbreak were indicted in the United States District Court in the Southern District of Florida. The male patient in our outbreak was sentenced to three years in federal prison for his role in the administration of unapproved and dangerous toxin to humans.

According to a report in the *Sun Sentinel*, a Fort Lauderdale newspaper, in 2007 the Florida couple in the outbreak settled a civil lawsuit against the supplier of the toxin, List Laboratories. A confidentiality agreement was signed.

In a bit of tragic irony, on October 26, 2009, plaintiff Bach A. McComb filed a lawsuit against List Biological Laboratories in the Florida Southern district Court for personal injury. It appears that this suit ended when List Laboratories filed for bankruptcy.

List Laboratories still maintains a business of selling a variety of toxins, including botulinum (website active November 3, 2015). They do have an application which must be completed for new customers requiring a description of business or university department, and a "brief description of the research planned with List's products." They still offer a vial of 100 µg of botulinum neurotoxin Type A Complex from Clostridium botulinum for $260.00. They state that "All orders must be received by 12:00 pm PST to be eligible for same day shipping." Their website claims:

> List Labs complies with federal regulations covering the possession and handling of bacteria and toxins. We have designed a laboratory to provide the appropriate containment to protect both laboratory workers and the environment. Documented procedures and a well-developed training program support operations compliant with regulations.
>
> List Labs is registered with the CDC Select Agents and Toxins Program for Tier 1 agents, and the staff is trained and experienced in BSL 3 large scale manufacturing. During more than thirty years of experience in working with toxins and bacteria, we have developed the necessary infrastructure to support manufacturing and shipping according to regulations. We can apply our knowledge to your project and help you develop an approach to compliance.

Suggested Reading

Chertow DS, Tan ES, Maslanka SE, et al. Botulism in 4 adults following cosmetic injections with an unlicensed, highly concentrated botulinum preparation. JAMA. 2006;206(20):2476–9.

Marcus SM. Reflections on the area of a patient severely poisoned by "rogue" botulinum toxin and rendered paralysed for a protracted hospital stay. Botulinum J. 2009;1(3):318–39.

Souayah N, Karim H, Kamin SS, et al. Severe botulism after focal injection of botulinum toxin. Neurology. 2006;67:1855–6.

Chapter 7
Strange Wind Blowing

These you may eat of all that are in the waters; all that have fins and scales, you may eat. But whatever does not have fins and scales, you shall not eat; it is unclean for you.
   —Deuteronomy 14:9–10.[1]

Fifty-five-year-old, semi-retired Jim Pallucci (pseudonym) had had one of those awful weeks in which nothing seemed to go right. He had put in eleven-hour days every day and still didn't seem to be getting anywhere at work. All week, he had just one thing in mind, meeting his nephew Robbie (pseudonym) on Saturday morning and fishing at his favorite spot off a nearby pier. Robbie, the seventeen-year-old son of Jim's sister, idolized him and looked forward to all the time Jim spent with him. The thought of the sun and salt air invigorated Jim and he was able to forge forward. The Palluccis were transplanted New Yorkers from Long Island. They moved to Florida with their parents when Jim was in high school and his sister had just started college. Jim recalled the times he and his father fished on the Long Island Sound. Those days, pulling in porgies and blowfish and occasionally blues, when they were running, were a fond memory and he hoped that Robbie would have memories such as these when he grew up.

The week dragged on and Jim was very tired when Friday night rolled around. He left work at 6:30 p.m. and pulled up to his condo at 7:15 p.m. On the weekends when he would spend time with Robbie, he usually went to his sister's house for dinner on Friday night, slept over, and spent the rest of the weekend playing side-kick to Robbie. Since his sister's divorce three years ago, he was the important male influence in Robbie's life. This Friday, however, the thought of dinner was surpassed by the need for sleep, and Jim decided to forgo the dinner at his sister's house. As soon as he reached home he popped a TV dinner in the microwave and called his sister to beg off. He spoke to Robbie, and told him that they were still on

---

[1] The Complete Jewish Bible, translated by Rabbi A. J. Rosenberg, Chabad.org. http://www.chabad.org/library/bible_cdo/aid/9978/jewish/Chapter-14.htm#v=9 (accessed 21 March 2016).

© Springer International Publishing AG 2017
S.M. Marcus, *Medical Toxicology: Antidotes and Anecdotes*,
DOI 10.1007/978-3-319-51029-3_7

for their fishing expedition and that he would pick him up bright and early in the morning. Robbie had never been fishing with him; in fact Robbie had only been fishing once before. He did have his father's fishing rod. Robbie was excited about trying it out.

Jim pulled off his tie, pushed off his shoes, opened the refrigerator, and pulled out a beer while the dinner was cooking. The cold brew felt wonderful to his parched throat and the taste was near perfection to him. He felt relaxation spread over his torso. The turkey dinner tasted nothing like his sister's roast turkey and had a consistency like silly putty, but it did fill him up enough to allow him to finish his beer and head for his bedroom. He debated on a shower, but decided to hit the bed instead. His head had hardly hit the pillow when he drifted off into slumberland.

The alarm roused him out of a deep sleep at 6:30 a.m. He had thirty minutes to shower, shave and make the three minute trip to pick up Robbie. His day off and he was already behind, what a laugh!

When he pulled his Chevy Tahoe into his sister's driveway, Robbie was already opening the garage door, fishing rod in hand all ready to hop into the car. Robbie's mother handed Jim a thermos of coffee and wished them good luck. Off they went, uncle and nephew, happy as larks, ready to spend the day on the pier hauling in a load of fish.

They arrived at the pier at 8:00 a.m. Already the pier was alive with fellow fishermen. It was a veritable rainbow of fishermen of all races and dressed in all types of fishing gear. Some had fancy fishing rods and reels, others simple cord lines dropped over the side. Jim and Robbie chose a spot near the end of the pier, set up their folding chairs, and introduced themselves to their fishing neighbors. Jim then baited Robbie's hook and they were off on their fishing adventure. An hour went by without even so much as a bite. They struck up conversation with the Adamses (pseudonym), a father and son who were fishing on their right, and the Petersons (pseudonym), a husband and wife who appeared to be in their mid-sixties and were fishing on their left. They shared tales of previous fishing trips. Suddenly Robbie's fishing rod started to pulsate: he had a bite. Carefully he reeled in his prize. When they got it up on the pier they looked in amazement, the creature had strange fins, like wings at the sides.

"That's a sea robin," stated Mr. Adams, "not worth much of anything. Better get the hook out of his mouth and throw him back." Robbie's face showed both extreme disappointment, and a bit of disgust at the prospect of putting his hands on the poor beast to extricate the hook. Jim helped him wrap the thrashing fish in a towel and pull out the hook. They threw it back as far as they could away from the pier, giggling all the time and hoping the stupid fish would not bite on Robbie's hook again.

Less than five minutes later, Robbie pulled in his first real catch. This time a ten-inch-long brown fish plopped onto the pier and immediately expanded to three times its size. Robbie was amazed at the sight of this object which first seemed to be a smallish fish but now appeared to be bigger than a softball but smaller than a basketball. "That's a blowfish," said Mrs. Adams. Mr. Adams added, "Throw him back too, they are poisonous." "Nonsense," replied Jim, "We eat them all the time. When I grew up in New York, everyone ate them. They even had fish bakes where you could get all you could eat for $10.00!" "Well I won't eat them," replied Mr. Adams. "I'll make you a deal," said Jim, "we will take all you can catch."[2]

It seemed as if fate had heard the statement, for in the next six hours, the Adamses, Jim, and Robbie had amassed a bucket of 100 blowfish. It was as if a school of fish stopped below the pier and developed a feeding frenzy around their fish lines. Their fishing buckets overflowed with dead fish in various stages of inflation.

True to their statements, the Adamses offered all of their catch to Jim and Robbie. Jim then taught Robbie how to clean the fish. Blowfish are an interesting fish; the skin is bumpy but there are no scales, so there is no need to clean the skin. The edible meat is found as two roughly cylindrical muscles running along the backbone. If one is careful, one can cut off the rest of the fish and pull back on the skin leaving the muscle attached to the backbone in a fillet. After a few false steps in the process, both Jim and Robbie managed to clean each one of the nearly 100 fish. They placed the fish back into a bucket of cool sea water and left the pier. On their way off of the pier they stopped at a convenient ice machine which seemed to be placed there just for them and they iced their catch.

On the drive back to Robbie's house, they laughed about their adventure. As they approached the house, reality sunk in; what were they going to do with nearly 100 blow fish fillets?

Robbie's mother was less than enthralled by the prospect of freezing the loot in her deep chest freezer. It would take a year to consume all of the fish. They had to figure out what to do.

A few phone calls later and the answer was apparent; they would pack up the frozen fish and Jim would distribute the fish to relatives: a cousin in Florida, another in North Carolina, and two in New Jersey. Jim had to make a business trip to New York City the following week and offered to transport some of the fish to his uncle in New Jersey. Jim's uncle and aunt were retired and loved fish. They expressed joy and the prospect of seeing Jim and receiving the fish.

Jim left Robbie and his mother at around 9 p.m. that night, secure in his plan to distribute their prize.

The following week the fish reached their destinations. In New Jersey, Joe and Marie (pseudonyms) defrosted the first 12 fillets. They planned a nice quiet dinner at home. Marie was planning on cooking the fish and making stew with the leftovers. As Marie cooked the fish, Joe set the table and cut up the vegetables. They had purchased some nice, pencil-thin asparagus from the local greengrocer to accent their fish meal. They sat down to the dinner table at 7:30 p.m. and both began eating the fish. It tasted wonderful and there was no hint at the dire consequences that were about to strike. Joe finished four of the fillets and Marie six before they both decided they had had enough. They began cleaning the table when Marie mentioned that her lips and tongue felt odd. Joe remarked that he was afraid to say anything, fearing that Marie would think he was nuts. They both agreed that the spices Marie had used must have affected them. By the time the dinner dishes were rinsed and placed into

---

[2]This dialogue was fabricated to describe the discussion regarding different "known" toxicities of blowfish in different locations.

the dishwasher, Marie was complaining of nausea and, barely five minutes later, started vomiting her meal into the toilet. Frightened, Joe picked up the telephone and called the local poison control center. The information specialist on duty asked if they had eaten any shellfish, to which Joe answered that he had eaten mussels several days ago, but none on the day of this experience. Marie between bouts of vomiting, yelled out to Joe that she had numbness spreading up her left arm. At this point the specialist suggested that Joe and Marie go to the nearest hospital emergency department.

I was watching one of my favorite mystery shows on television when the telephone rang. It was Man Yee Wong (we called her Mae), a pharmacist working as one of the poison information specialists calling me to discuss a case. She received a telephone call regarding a woman and her husband, both in their sixties. They reported they had each eaten frozen blowfish that the husband's brother gave them. The brother had been in Florida and had been fishing off of a pier in Florida. He caught a bumper crop of blowfish. He gutted, cleaned, and filleted the fish and then froze them. On coming north, he brought the frozen fish in a cooler with him. He made a few stops along the way to drop off fish with friends and relatives before finishing his northbound trip in New Jersey. The husband and wife ate about six pieces of the blowfish each. Within a half an hour both of them developed numbness and tingling of their lips and tongue and the woman started vomiting. Mae referred them into the hospital and, at the time of the call to me, they were in the hospital emergency room. Dr. Dan Bergio (pseudonym) was the attending physician in the emergency department that night and requested to speak to me. Dr. Bergio confirmed the complaints and symptoms expressed via telephone with Mae. The numbness had spread to the rest of their faces and down their arms. In addition, the female complained of some chest discomfort.

I explained to Dr. Bergio that I had really never heard of East Coast blowfish causing any problems. I mentioned that when I was growing up, during summers on Long Island I had both caught and eaten many blowfish and never experienced any of the couple's symptoms. The most common form of fish-related food poisoning is due to ciguatera toxin, which does produce similar neurological findings. At the time of this case presentation, I was under the impression that blowfish found on the East Coast of the United States were not associated with such a poisoning. The only blowfish poisoning that I was aware of at the time was that from eating fugu.

Fugu is one of the most notorious dishes in Japanese cuisine. It is Japanese delicacy derived from blowfish, in Japan more often called puffer fish, and whose toxin, tetrodotoxin, can actually be fatal. Fugu is frequently served as sashimi. But there are restaurants which serve fugu soup, stew, deep fried, or baked. Unfortunately for any hapless victim, the toxin is heat stable, so cooking will not deactivate it. It is estimated that over twenty thousand tons of fugu are consumed in Japan every year.

The ingestion of fugu dates probably from antiquity. Some believe that the biblical warning about not eating fish that lack fins and scales refer to the Red Sea blowfish. In medieval times, the Tokugawa shogunate banned blowfish consumption. There is copious folklore related to fugu. There are sonnets and poems written about its use. There is even a fugu museum in Osaka. The owner of the museum is reported to have said: "Human beings are funny. They want to eat what is forbidden. The history of blowfish is the history of prohibition by authorities. If blowfish weren't poisonous, they might not be so popular."[3]

In Japan, since 1958, fugu chefs must obtain a special license to prepare and sell fugu. The chefs serve an apprenticeship which may last several years. There is a licensing examination which must then be passed before the chef is allowed to prepare fugu for the public. The examination consists of a written test, a fish-identification test, and a practical test, preparing and eating the fish. Reportedly only about 35% of the applicants pass. The information as to the fate of those who fail is not reported.[4] Restaurants in Japan are allowed to sell pre-packaged fugu prepared by a licensed practitioner.

Tetrodotoxin blocks the opening of the sodium channel, that pathway through which sodium rapidly moves into the cell while potassium leaves the cell and thus causes it to become active. In muscle cells the blockade will essentially cause the paralysis of the muscle. It is estimated that tetrodotoxin is over 1200 times as lethal as cyanide. If the muscles affected are those that provide breathing, the individual will die a respiratory death. Each year there are between 70 and 100 deaths from eating fugu worldwide.

Never having heard of a neurotoxin in eastern blowfish, we asked that the fish be identified, and Dr. Bergio replied that the couple continued to insist that the fish were blowfish. Having never heard of U.S. blowfish causing such neurological symptoms, I continued to believe that the identification had been wrong and that the couple had in fact contracted ciguatera toxin from eating fish contaminated with that toxin (see Chap. 2). The therapy for ciguatera poisoning, although not proven effective in any clinical trials, has been anecdotally reported as being helpful at relieving the symptoms and is relatively benign. It was elected to treat the husband and wife with mannitol, a non-absorbable sugar which is said to pull toxins out of the blood through the kidneys and into the urine. Both of them received an infusion of mannitol.

The husband's symptoms disappeared very rapidly after the infusion of mannitol. His wife continued to complain of tingling around her mouth and then she developed discomfort on the left side of her chest. More worrisome, she developed a rapid heart rate of 109 beats per minute, and her blood pressure increased to 160/70. She was treated with a medication called Nitropaste, a brand of topically applied nitroglycerin, in an attempt to both lower her blood pressure and relieve her chest discomfort. Over the ensuing two to three hours, she developed weakness of her extremities and decreased ability to breathe. When she was found to be breathing so poorly that she was retaining carbon dioxide and her inspiratory volume

[3] Asif Khan, "Fugu: This Fish Dish Can Kill You, Recommended Only for the Brave and the Suicidal," 28 April 2016, Inquisitr, http://www.inquisitr.com/3041539/fugu-this-fish-dish-can-kill-you-recommended-only-for-the-brave-and-the-suicidal/ (accessed 13 June 2016).

[4] Steve Lohr, "ONE MAN'S FUGU IS ANOTHER'S POISON" NY Times, 29 November 1981. http://www.nytimes.com/1981/11/29/travel/one-man-s-fugu-is-another-s-poison.html (accessed 28 July 2016).

dropped to 20% of the normal for her age and size, she was electively intubated. A tube was inserted into her windpipe through her mouth and this was attached to a mechanical respirator to keep her breathing artificially. She was given sedation and kept on the ventilator for forty-eight hours. During that time, her muscle tone returned and her symptoms completely disappeared. She was taken off of the ventilator and the tube removed. By forty eight hours after the admission, both the husband and wife were totally asymptomatic. They told us that there was left over fish in their home freezer. We reached out to the local health department and the local health officer went to their home and obtained the still frozen leftover fish for analysis. At our request, the fish was kept in a biological deep freezer until we could find someone to analyze it.

After their recovery, we interviewed the husband and wife and the brother to clarify the type of fish and where the fish had been obtained. The brother confirmed that, in late February, he was fishing off of a pier in Florida, and it was there that he caught the fish. He remarked about how many blowfish he was able to catch. He gutted, cleaned, filleted, and froze the fish after catching them. He stated that the fish never thawed while under his care; he kept the fish frozen in his freezer until his drive back north. During his drive, the fish were kept frozen in a cooler in his car. He made several stops on the trip north to distribute his catch to friends and relatives on the route. We suggested that he reach out to all of those to whom he gave fish and that no one should eat any of the fish. We requested that any remaining fish be sent to us frozen, for analysis. We asked the local health department of the husband and wife's town to obtain the left over fish and keep that frozen for analysis as well.

The center staff then attempted to find a laboratory to analyze the fish. We were unsuccessful at that time, and requested that the samples be kept frozen by the health officer. Wondering if there were any other cases like ours, considering the number of fish reportedly pulled from that pier that day, I contacted the executive director of the American Association of Poison Control Centers to see if there had been any reports of severe neurological symptoms associated with food poisoning during the months prior to our test cases. Unfortunately, the association's computers were tied up at the time working with the information for its annual report, and I was told it would take some time to do a look back. Considering that we only had these two cases and we did not know whether they represented a wider public health problem, we elected not to pursue the look back with the national data program further.

Almost a month later I was awakened at five a.m. by Nancy DeMar, one of the information specialists at the New Jersey Poison Center. She was calling me to get my advice about a sixty-year-old man that was in an Emergency Department. The day before his presentation he ate a breakfast of blowfish. Soon after eating the blowfish he developed dizziness but ignored the symptoms. He ate more of the blowfish for lunch and developed weakness and dizziness and developed pins and needle sensation in all of his extremities. As the day progressed the symptoms became more profound, so he went to the emergency department. When seen he complained of being very dizzy, had difficulty walking, and demonstrated loss of coordination in his upper and lower extremities. On his physical examination, he was found to have high blood pressure with a systolic of 203 and a diastolic of 94; the remainder of his physical examination and laboratory evaluation was normal. We requested that a urine sample be obtained and be frozen. He was treated with intravenous fluids and improved over the next few hours. He was admitted for observation overnight and discharged asymptomatic the following morning.

We were able to obtain family contact information. I asked my associate Bruce Ruck, Pharm.D., to help me obtain further information. Dr. Ruck reached out to the patient's wife at around 11 a.m. in the morning. He obtained the information that the fish had been purchased in a retail seafood store in their local community. Ruck called the seafood store to confirm that it was in fact blowfish that the gentleman had purchased from them. Dr. Ruck then asked where the seafood store had obtained the fish. The seafood store owner explained that he got it from his usual wholesaler and gave the name and phone number of the wholesaler to him. Dr. Ruck was able to reach the wholesaler and found that the wholesaler had purchased the fish from the Fulton Fish Market which had recently relocated to the Bronx, New York. When Ruck reached the vendor at the Fulton Fish Market, he learned that the fish had been purchased from a Florida crabber and was able to obtain the name of the crabber. Ruck was able to contact the crabber. In a discussion with the crabber, Dr. Ruck learned that it is common to find a blowfish in crab traps. They are trapped and they are a nuisance fish. This time though, rather than simply throwing the fish back into the sea, the crabber decided that he would try to parlay it into making more profit by cleaning the fish and bringing the fish to market with his crabs. When questioned further it turned out that the crab traps that were used and trapped these blowfish were all within proximity of the exact same pier that the brother of the first cases did his fishing. It was obvious to us that we had an outbreak of a strange neurological type of poison from blowfish and, further, that the source of these contaminated fish was the fishing pier in Florida.

This circumstance both intrigued and frightened us. A quick review of the literature again revealed no significant reports of U.S. blowfish-related neurotoxins toxicity. Were we dealing with a new disease or a terrorist threat? Luckily, by then we had found a researcher in Nova Scotia, Mike Quilliam of the Marine Biosciences National Research Council. Dr. Quilliam was intrigued by the clinical presentation of the first couple and agreed to help us by analyzing the fish. He explained that he had developed an assay for tetratotoxin and other marine neurotoxins. When we explained that we had another individual, he was even more intrigued. He agreed to do the analysis for us gratis, as long as we paid for the shipment of the fish.

We received a call from Dr. Quilliam about two weeks later. Liquid chromographic-tandem mass spectrometric analysis of the uneaten fish samples failed to reveal any tetrodotoxin. Dr. Quilliam's lab was able to identify the presence of the paralytic shellfish poison saxitoxin, and two analogs, N-sulfocarbamoylsaxitoxin and decarbamoylsaxitoxin. A sample of the same fish was also submitted to the United States Food and Drug Administration's laboratory in Queens, New York, for analysis. That laboratory did not have an assay for that specific toxin, but did confirm the presence of a sodium-blocking toxin by cell bioassay. This confirmed the toxin as saxitoxin, as Dr. Quilliam's laboratory determined.

Saxitoxin, like tetrodotoxin, is heat stable. It cannot be destroyed by either cooking or freezing. It is produced by the dinoflagellate, *Gymnodinium catenatum*. The dinoflagellates multiply, bloom, in the water. Water-siphoning shellfish, principally mollusks such as clams, scallops and mussels siphon many hundreds of gallons of water though their filtering system every day. They filter out organisms to feed on and in the process absorb any toxin which accompanies them. The toxin then accumulates in the filtering system and in the muscle of the mollusks. Blowfish, also known as puffer fish, are known to eat mollusks and then "bio-amplify" and "bio-accumulate" the toxin in their muscles. The quanidinium moiety of the toxin enters the voltage-gated sodium channel and the imidazole ring then lodges in the opening of the channel leaving the rest of the molecule literally blocking the channel. The rapid movement of sodium through this channel is necessary for the propagation of neural impulses and contraction of muscle. The outcome of such blockage by this toxin is muscle paralysis. A mutation in the protein sequence of the sodium channel in the puffer fish, renders the sodium channel of the puffer resistant to the toxin.

There is no specific treatment for the poisoning. Physicians can only treat the victims symptomatically, although some have suggested using high concentrations of sodium in an effort to force the sodium channel open.

Eventually a look back for cases reported to poison centers over the previous months, combined with active surveillance for cases in hospital emergency departments and health departments' foodborne illness complaint logs, revealed a total of thirteen cases in three states, New Jersey, Virginia, and Florida.

How or why this toxin appeared in the puffer fish in this region remains a question. There are over 100 species of pufferfish worldwide and nine which exist in the waters off of Florida. Southern puffer fish have been increasing in population over the past decade. It is possible that this has occurred as part of the coastal water warming trend from the effects of global warming. The southern puffer fish caught by Jim Pallucci in Florida have been in that area for years, but were never previously implicated in previous fish poisoning events.

Shortly after the discovery of these cases, the New Jersey Department of Health and Senior Services issued a health alert calling for citizens to cease eating any puffer fish originating in the Titusville, Florida area. Soon after, the FDA issued a health advisory on puffer fish caught in this area. The Florida Department of Health, in collaboration with the Florida Department of Agriculture and Consumer Services posted warnings on the pier to cease fishing for such fish off of the pier and to release any caught.

Suggested Reading

Hammond R, Bodager D, Jackow G, et al. Update neurologic illness associated with eating florida pufferfish, 2002. Morb Mortal Wkly Rep. 2002;51(19):414–6.
Wolf G, Blumenstock J, Rose SR, et al. Neurologic illness associated with eating florida pufferfish, 2002. Morb Mortal Wkly Rep. 2002;51(15):321–3.

Chapter 8
Bubbles in the Toilet Water

According to Wikipedia, flat bread has been made since the Neolithic age.[1] Archeological evidence of its existence dates back at least seven thousand years. It is thought that these flat breads morphed into "pizza" sometime at the end of the first millennium. Some historians state that the existence of pizza as a widely sold food dates back to the early sixteenth century in Naples. That bread was not made with tomatoes until after Europeans returned from the Americas with the fruit in the late sixteenth century. Tomatoes are in the nightshade family. Some think of "deadly nightshade" when they hear that term. In fact, some believe that Europeans did not look upon the tomato as edible until they were shown by Americans it is safe and delicious. By the late eighteenth century, the bread topped with tomato sauce and cheese had become popular in Italy and became a "tourist attraction." With the mass migration of immigrants to the United States at the turn of the twentieth century, Italian immigrants brought their dish with them to the "new world." Inexpensive to make, it became very popular and it did not take long for pizza to spread first to Italian American communities and then to most of the country. It is probable that the first commercial pizza restaurant opened in New York's Little Italy. As the Italian population expanded and prospered, it ventured into the greener pastures of New Jersey. We know of the existence of pizza in Trenton, New Jersey, as early as 1910, when Joe's Tomato Pies opened, followed closely by Papa's Tomato Pies in 1912.

Pizza remained a favorite of Italian Americans and little known to others until after the Second World War. American troops in Italy became "addicted" to pizza and upon return precipitated the further growth of the pizza industry.

Some say that the state pie of New Jersey is the pizza pie. New Jersey prides itself on its unique style of thin pizza. Although no two pies are ever exactly the same, the distinctive "Jersey flavor" is evident with every bite. Every town in this

---

[1] Wikipedia History of pizza. https://en.wikipedia.org/wiki/History_of_pizza. Accessed 22 March 2016.

© Springer International Publishing AG 2017
S.M. Marcus, *Medical Toxicology: Antidotes and Anecdotes*,
DOI 10.1007/978-3-319-51029-3_8

state of 540 individual communities has at least one or two pizza-producing restaurants or storefront pizza parlors. They are extremely convenient places to drop in, grab a slice or two and a drink for lunch or a snack, and get on your way.

Renato Debellonia, a physician trained in Italy at the University of Bologna, had just recently come on duty as the poison information specialist at the New Jersey Poison Information Education System. It was just after 2 p.m., after he had his lunch of Italian salami on Italian bread with mozzarella cheese and sweet peppers, when he received a telephone call from a pizza restaurant describing an unusual event. Five businessmen had come to the restaurant for lunch. They ordered two pizzas to be split between them and each had a pasta dish. One was a cheese pizza the other was a pepperoni pizza. Each man had a different pasta dish; all had pasta which was made with a red sauce but with different meats. Three of the men ordered sodas and two ordered iced tea. While discussing their business they each consumed their share of pizza. About a half an hour after finishing their meals, while still in the restaurant, they began to complain of stomachache and three of the five began vomiting shortly thereafter. The owner of the restaurant, aware that he had the potential outbreak of food borne illness within his restaurant, called the poison center for help. Debellonia suggested that they be allowed to drink just sips of fluid once they stopped vomiting. He suggested that, if they had any ginger ale in the store that the ginger might help calm their stomachs. He added that they would need to seek the services of their family physician or emergency room if the vomiting continued. There were other patrons in the restaurant at the same time and no one else became ill. In fact, the owner and three workers were fine, remarking they also ate pizza made the same day. In time, the three men who became sick recovered and with the two men that didn't become sick, the five men left the store.

Debellonia contacted the local health department to investigate the outbreak in the restaurant. He maintained contact with the owner of the restaurant to ensure that there were no further cases. Before terminating the conversation, Debellonia conducted a careful food intake history. He attempted to form a table of the foods that each of the patrons of the restaurant had eaten that day and what happened to them after they ate. He set up a table with those who became ill in one column, listing everything they ate or drank, and in a second column the things that people who did not become ill ate and drank. He determined that the types of pasta that all five individuals ate as well as the pizza were the same; there was no difference between the food of those that became sick and those that stayed well. It became obvious that the three individuals that developed abdominal pain and vomiting all had ordered "fountain sodas"—that is, sodas that were made from the soda machine within the restaurant. The other two ordered bottled iced tea. The only thing that Debellonia could find to divide those who became sick from those who stayed well was the fountain soda. Other individuals had been in the restaurant that day and had eaten pizza without any event. Interestingly, there had been no other individuals that had fountain soda that entire day. All of the previous customers that day had ordered bottled or canned sodas or other drinks. The owner mentioned that it could not be a problem with the fountain soda, since the soda machine had not been working properly and was serviced by a contractor the day before the events. The service contractor replaced the coil inside of the machine that carries water through the refrigerating portion of the machine so that cold soda would be dispensed.

Full questioning of employees of the restaurant revealed that they had noticed something peculiar in the men's room that morning. They reported that the water in the toilet seemed to be bubbling as if it was soda water. They also noticed that the water coming out of the cold water taps seemed to be carbonated. Debellonia suggested that they shut down the soda machine and stop using it for dispensing of drinks. He suggested that they call the repairman back and limit the sale of drinks to packaged sodas and drinks. The rest of the day was busy at the restaurant with no repeat of abdominal pain or vomiting. All of the customers drank bottled or canned beverage, and nobody consumed anything more coming out of the machine. They sold their usual pizza and pasta without incident.

Food related illness is a common phenomenon. The threats to the food supply are great and include biological agents, bacteria, mycological (fungal) agents, and viruses, as well as non-biological agents such as metals, chemicals, and pesticides. Often the relationship is missed by the victim, and even his or her physician. We have all come down with the "I must have eaten something that disagreed with me." Closely behind that comment is "I guess I ate, or drank, too much," or "That food was just too rich for me." Usually, even if the victim (as in this case) develops vomiting and or diarrhea, he or she becomes better, since most exposure symptoms are self-limited, and no one pursues any form of investigation. That is unfortunate because those initial cases could be the onset of a more widespread illness. Because of that possibility, food poisonings are generally reportable to the health department. In New Jersey any such food poisoning is reportable to the health department of the town in which the victim lives, interestingly, not to the health department responsible for the sanitary conditions of the restaurant.

Generally, the time between ingestion and the onset of symptoms as well as the type of food ingested gives an investigator an insight into the possible cause of the food poisoning. It is vital to keep surveillance and preventive efforts high in order to avoid widespread illness. It is similarly important to identify a potential outbreak early, analyze the data involved, make a presumptive diagnosis of cause, and attempt to both mitigate any illness and terminate any potential exposure. Every outbreak begins with a single "index" case. Any encounter with such an index case is an opportunity to make an early diagnosis and perhaps terminate the outbreak. Thus it is important to develop a plan to use to approach any cluster of illnesses.

The United States Food and Drug Administration periodically publishes a book, *The Bad Bug Book*,[2] which discusses the various infectious agents causing food borne illnesses. This guide serves as a useful "how to" manual for evaluating a case of food poisoning and searching for a possible cause.

Patients with food borne illnesses generally present with gastrointestinal symptoms and signs. Early signs usually consist of nausea, vomiting, abdominal pain,

---

[2] Bad Bug Book (Second Edition) Foodborne Pathogenic Microorganisms and Natural Toxins Handbook http://www.fda.gov/Food/FoodborneIllnessContaminants/CausesOfIllnessBadBugBook/ accessed 22 March 2016.

and diarrhea. Once a foodborne illness is suspected, important clues include: (1) incubation period—that is, time between exposure and development of symptoms; (2) presenting symptoms and signs; (3) population involved in the outbreak; (4) duration of the illness; and (5) the ingestion of common potential sources of food poisoning, such as raw or improperly cooked foods, foods left out for extended periods of time, high-risk foods such as eggs, shellfish, soft cheeses, and unpasteurized milk, cider, or cheeses.

An individual who develops gastrointestinal symptoms within a very short time after the exposure has likely been exposed to a metal contamination. Metals are extremely irritating to the gastric mucous membranes (stomach linings). Such metals as arsenic, copper, thallium, or zinc contamination usually produce vomiting within minutes of the exposure. Shellfish—specifically, bivalve mollusks—siphon and filter large amounts of water through their gill structures. Anything contaminating the filtered water can be caught in the filter mechanism. In this manner they can become contaminated with various metals, from arsenic to lead, mercury, and cadmium. The ingestion of such shellfish can then produce early onset symptoms and signs. Additionally, collected blood or urine from individuals who ingest shellfish can give astoundingly frightening results when analyzed for such metals as arsenic and mercury. Luckily for the human ingesting the mollusks, these metals are converted by the mollusk into an organic form, which, although potentially causing local irritation and vomiting, is not thought to produce any systemic or lasting effects. Many kitchens have copper pots and pans used in cooking. The copper is used for the backbone of the pots and pans, because of the ease and uniformity with which heat is spread in the copper. They are generally "tinned" where the food is cooked to avoid contamination of the food with the copper. Occasionally, there is a scratch through the tin allowing the food to come into contact with the copper as it is being prepared and contaminating the food. The copper in the food can be extremely irritating, producing abdominal distress very rapidly after its consumption. Soaps and other cleaning solutions may be inadequately rinsed off of the cooking or serving equipment and contamination with these can lead to rapid onset of symptoms. I remember an event in which I was part of a group dining out at a very fancy restaurant that became ill shortly after leaving the restaurant. When we compared notes as to what we all ate and drank, those of us who became ill all had coffee, and those who had tea did not. We then spoke to the restaurant's sanitarian and tracked down the probable source of our illness: the coffee service had been scrubbed clean with a commercial cleaning agent that day in preparation for the following day's celebration of New Years' Eve. He postulated that the serving equipment might not have been adequately rinsed before it was used to serve us.

Exposures to high concentrations of nitrites—as in contaminated water from boilers, or the mistaken use of sodium nitrite (saltpeter, also called corning salt) instead of sodium chloride (table salt)—can produce rapid onset abdominal distress and vomiting (see Chap. 1 in this book).

Various toxins derived from fish can present with symptoms very early but often are not immediately recognized as foodborne. Scombroid fish poisoning occurs from the ingestion of fish, primarily in the scombroid family (such as tuna, bluefish, sardines, anchovies, and mackerel), that have not been kept adequately cold after catching. The use of the "long line" in trolling for fish can produce the circumstances which lead to this exposure. A "long line" is a steel cable which may be as long as a mile long which has hundreds of fish hooks attacked and with bait on each hook. The line is released and the boat "trolls" an area for hours before the line is reeled in. It is thus possible that a fish can be caught early in a day and not harvested back onto the ship for many hours. Drowned by the trolling boat, the fish may float closer to the surface where the warmer water encourages the growth of bacteria on the skin of the fish (one of the most commonly involved is morganella morganii), which convert the amino acid histidine into histamine. The hapless diner eating the fish has an exaggerated histamine reaction with hives and even broncho-constriction, interference with breathing. Such fish as tuna, bluefish, and others can become so intoxicated. As with other fish toxins, scombroid is heat stable, colorless, and tasteless thus the risk exists if fish are not kept at cold enough temperatures and continues even if the fish is cooked properly. I had my own personal experience with this toxin in my hospital cafeteria. The director of the cafeteria asked me to try a new brand of tuna he was considering to serve in the hospital. Within fifteen minutes I developed flushing of my face, sweating, dizziness, and urticaria (hives). I was rushed to the emergency room by my associates thinking that the next would be respiratory embarrassment. I was given a dose of diphenhydramine (Benadryl) and the symptoms cleared over the next hour. The cafeteria decided not to serve the fish.

A bacteria which produces toxins, so-called preformed toxin, contaminating the food or a bacteria which produces toxin rapidly and then contaminates food may produce an illness with a short incubation period. The technique of precooking rice and keeping it in a warming container, hot enough for it to stay warm, but not hot enough to kill bacteria, can produce the right environment for the bacteria bacillus cereus to grow and release its toxin. Reheating the rice, as in making fried rice, then produces the potential for illness. Staphylococcus contamination of meats, potato and egg salads, cream pastries, etc., produces a preformed toxin with a short incubation period of one to six hours. The illness is generally characterized by a sudden onset of severe nausea, vomiting, and abdominal cramping pain with or without diarrhea within four to six hours of a meal which includes the suspect foods.

Slightly more delayed can be poisoning from various mushrooms, the worst of which, the amanita mushroom, can cause significant liver and kidney damage. This happens when immigrants, used to picking wild mushrooms in their native land, mistake wild mushrooms in this country for those they are used to and end up with toxicity from the toxins in our wild mushrooms. There are other forms of toxic wild mushrooms; some produce psychedelic effects, others an interaction with alcoholic beverages producing severe headaches. There is also a form of wild mushroom that can damage kidneys. There is an old saying: "There are old mushroom pickers, and there are bold mushroom pickers. There are no old, bold mushroom pickers."

Onset starting at twelve hours or more after ingestion, associated with fever, is often from contamination with the bacterium streptococcus which can also produce an associated sore throat. Infections with parasites organisms, such as amoebae and other micro-organisms and worms, generally have longer latent periods.

Back to the restaurant, a repairman came to look at the soda machine. He found that the internal stainless-steel water coil used inside of the machine, which transported bubbling soda water through the refrigeration system producing cold soda, had been incorrectly replaced with a less expensive, copper coil. The water intake to the machine had also been repaired incorrectly. When the machine was reattached it was attached without a back flow valve. Without the backflow valve, carbonated water from the machine could back flow from the machine into the restaurant's general water supply. Carbonated water had seeped back into all of the cold water within the restaurant, hence the appearance of carbonated water in the toilets and in the sinks when the cold water tap was turned on.

Carbonated water results from the bubbling of carbon dioxide into water. Much of the gaseous carbon dioxide stays in the non-dissolved form and forms the characteristic bubbles of soda water. Some of the carbon dioxide becomes dissolved in the water producing carbonic acid. Carbonic acid is a weak acid. Once absorbed into the body by ingestion, it exists in physiological solutions in an equilibrium that exists between a bicarbonate ion and a hydrogen ion. This equilibrium is found throughout nature. The body handles carbonic acid through an enzyme called carbonic anhydrous and breaks it down into bicarbonate and hydrogen. In soda the typical temperature and pressure (of a closed container, bottle or can) keeps a high concentration of undissolved CO_2 producing the bubbles, but there is some dissolution and hence carbonic acid which makes the water acid in nature and contributes to both the sour and sparkling taste of the drinks. Carbonic acid is capable of dissolving metals that it comes in contact with. Thus, when lying in contact with copper tubing, carbonic acid has the potential to dissolve significant amounts of copper into the water. The degree of such contamination will depend on the length of time the water containing the acid stays in contact with the copper. The knowledge of the potential to find copper contaminating the water in soda machines has been known for over one hundred years. That contamination may occur within the machine. The contamination of the rest of the water in a building because of a non-functional backflow valve has only been reported in the last few decades.

In looking at the overall water system at the restaurant and in the rest of the building housing the restaurant, the majority of the cold water pipes were made from copper tubing. Copper tubing is a frequently used substance for water pipes. It replaced galvanized metal and lead pipes over the past hundred years or so. Generally thought of as safe and easy to work with copper rapidly became the plumbing metal of choice. Copper tubing is supplied in certain lengths which are then soldered together with joints that form a waterproof and leak proof seam out between lengths of copper tubing. Until recently, the major metal in solder was lead. Water that sits in the piping could theoretically "pickup" some copper or even lead from the solder used in the joints of the copper tubing and add such metals to the water. If one drinks the water that has been sitting in the pipe for some time one can get exposed to significant quantities of these metals. Examination of the water in the restaurant found that the water supply was indeed contaminated with copper. During the repairs of the soda machine, the input and output of the machine became mixed up and carbonated water was being spread through the regular water supply of the building.

Thus carbonated water filled all of the copper tubing throughout the restaurant, including the toilets, hence the bubbles in the water in the toilets. Sometimes when soda dispensing machines are repaired, the repairperson forgets and uses a copper coil inside of the machine when he or she should have used stainless steel. This results in carbon dioxide bubbled into the water and producing a high concentration of carbonic acid. There have been many reports in the literature of similar events occurring in restaurants for the very same reason as occurred in this circumstance.

There is controversy over the long-term effects of drinking carbonated water. It is theoretically possible to drink enough carbonated water, and hence carbonic acid, to change the body's configuration as far as the body's acidity. As the body becomes more acid, the potential exists for the loss of bone density from the bones of the body as well as the loss of enamel from the teeth as the carbonic acid in the mouth leaches out some enamel. These potential health effects are far different than the effects of copper on the gastrointestinal mucosa.

Suggested Reading

CETCIMAGAZINE. Carbon dioxide leak in soda machines. http://www.critical-environment. com/blog/carbon-dioxide-co2-leak-in-soda-machines/. Accessed 3 July 2013.
Spitalny KC, Brondum J, Vogt RL, et al. Drinking water-induced copper intoxication in a Vermont family. Pediatrics. 1984;74:1103–6 .http://pediatrics.aapublications.org/content/74/6/1103

Chapter 9
Making Ice Cream the Modern Way

During weekends and summer months, many colleges and museums either lease out their classrooms and laboratories for enrichment programs or run their own programs. The program involved in this case was at a New Jersey university that had been running such a program for many years. This year's summer session had been going on for several days. The concept was to make science fun. When I heard about the experiment that led to the call to the poison center, I remembered as a child watching the television show *Mr. Wizard*. In that show Don Herbert, the "wizard," exposed his viewers to science in a totally painless, educational, and fun way. The show was somewhat formulaic, but that was the standard for that era; a neighbor, his assistant for that show, would come over to see Mr. Wizard and they would then embark on an exploration of some scientific phenomenon. While many children were entertained by Howdy Doody and the Lone Ranger, many of us became fascinated with the prospect of doing scientific experiments at home, following the directions of Mr. Wizard and his assistant. The amazing thing about the original show, which ran from 1951 through 1965, was the ability to make the most mundane experiments look like fun and to titillate the minds of the watchers to go further and learn more about the subjects presented.

I was not alone in my fascination with Mr. Wizard. According to his obituary: "During the 1960s and '70s, about half the applicants to Rockefeller University in New York, where students work toward doctorates in science and medicine, cited Mr. Wizard when asked how they first became interested in science."[1]

I graduated from college midyear. The college's policy was that one had to graduate upon completing 128 credits. I left college and went to work for New York Medical College. It was in the early days of learning about receptors, and I was busy looking at cardiac adrenergic receptors (those associated with the fight-or-flight response of the body). We would dose animals with rauwolfia, an alkaloid of plant

---

[1] Goldstein R. (2007 June 13). Don Herbert, 'Mr. Wizard' to Science Buffs, Dies at 89. New York Times. Access on line at: http://www.nytimes.com/2007/06/13/arts/13herbert.html?_r=0 (accessed on March 23, 2016).

© Springer International Publishing AG 2017
S.M. Marcus, *Medical Toxicology: Antidotes and Anecdotes*,
DOI 10.1007/978-3-319-51029-3_9

origin, which depletes the adrenergic receptors of their inherent catecholamines (epinephrine and nor-epinephrine, the actual chemicals involved in the apparent stimulatory effects). This allowed us to study the cardiac glycosides and how they affect the cardiac rhythm or force of contraction. We would sacrifice the rauwolfia-treated animals and remove their hearts for study. Rather than homogenize them in a blender, we found it easier and more efficient to drop the hearts into liquid nitrogen and then smash them in a device which essentially pulverized them into small enough pieces to allow for solubilizing them.

Liquid nitrogen is made by fractionating nitrogen from the air—it normally represents 78% of the air we breathe—in a process termed fractionalization distillation. The result of such a process, the gas placed under pressure becomes a liquid. At normal atmospheric pressure, liquid nitrogen boils at -195.79 °C (77 K; -320 °F). Heat is required to convert any liquid to a gas, as is observed when boiling water on a stove; this is called the heat of vaporization. When liquid nitrogen converts from liquid to gas, it absorbs heat from its surroundings and becomes a cryogenic fluid that can cause rapid freezing on contact with tissue. Exposure of living tissue can produce a burn, also known as a frost bite.

We had to be very careful how we stored, poured, and used the liquid nitrogen. It was stored in specially constructed conical containers which were both insulated and constructed in such a way as to maintain both the low temperature of the liquid nitrogen and the pressure inside the container, to keep the nitrogen in its liquid state. I wore insulated gloves when handling the equipment and the liquid nitrogen. When I poured it, it rapidly became a gaseous cloud and the chamber that I poured it into, which contained the heart muscle, froze rapidly to a solid. I was always very careful to avoid any contact with my skin to avoid developing frost-bite.

Returning to the case involving a dangerous exposure to liquid nitrogen it happened during a summer high school student enrichment program. The day was a beautiful August Friday. At midday, a class of "gifted" high school students were attending a special program at the university. The class that day was on using liquid nitrogen to make "instant ice cream." This procedure shortens the process of making ice cream from possibly hours to minutes. It is also exciting to watch. In addition to the display, the procedure is said to produce an exceptionally smooth ice cream and the flash freezing avoids the possibility of ice crystals forming, making the cream ever so much smoother than regular ice cream. You simply drop cream and flavoring into the liquid nitrogen while stirring and within seconds, voilà, you have ice cream.

A popular demonstration used in these science demonstrations often includes the "Leiden frost" effect. The Leiden frost effect is the generation of an "insulating" vapor barrier between the liquid nitrogen and skin that slows the transfer of the cold from the liquid nitrogen to any tissue such as the tongue or the inside of the mouth and thus prevents burns when liquid nitrogen is poured onto the palm of the hand, or dropped onto the tongue.

The teacher demonstrated that he could pour a little liquid nitrogen onto his hand and not get burned. But if he had closed his hand or poured a larger amount of the liquid nitrogen onto his hand, he would have been "burned," creating a frost bite. The "Leiden frost" effect is also seen at high temperatures; for example, when cold water droplets are dropped into a hot frying pan and the droplets bounce around the surface of the frying pan instead of boiling away. The teacher dropped a few drops of liquid nitrogen on his tongue, producing a plume of smoke but no burn.

In the classroom science experiment, the group then observed the demonstration of ice cream preparation with the use of liquid nitrogen for rapid cooling. The teacher demonstrated that mixing the cream and flavoring in a ball and then pouring in small amounts of liquid nitrogen while rapidly stirring with a wooden spoon produced delicious ice cream that the entire class shared.

The poison center received a telephone call that a teenage male having seen the demonstration of the "Leiden frost" effect, thought it would be "cool" to see what would happen if he swallowed liquid nitrogen. He was reported to have ingested about "half a cup" of liquid nitrogen about thirty minutes prior to the call to the poison center. The teenager then collapsed and suffered a seizure. Emergency medical services was called and responded. He was transported to an emergency department (ED) where he was at the time of the call to the poison center. The report from the ED said he was sweating, had a rapid heart rate, his blood pressure was high, and he was taking "deep breaths" and was having difficulty speaking. The ED doctor and the toxicologist on call had a discussion that this child should be taken to the operating room as quickly as possible, as it was very likely that the ingestion of this amount of liquid nitrogen would cause significant burns (frost burns can be as bad as heat burns) in the esophagus and stomach and the rapidly expanding nitrogen would most likely result in significant injury to the stomach and other organs. Luckily for the planned intervention, the on-call anesthesiologist had just returned from a continuing medical education program where they discussed liquid nitrogen and the fact that the expansion from the liquid to gas results in an enormous increase in volume. The gas:liquid volume ratio for nitrogen is about 700 to 1, the ingestion of 30 mL (approximately one ounce) of liquid nitrogen could result in the generation of several liters of nitrogen gas. The anesthesiologist agreed that, if this occurred in the stomach, the increase in pressure within the stomach from the expanding gas volume would rapidly lead to the point in which the stomach could no longer expand any further. The result would be a perforation of the stomach, literally an explosion. Fearing that the teenager would have difficulty breathing, an airway tube was inserted into his trachea and he was placed on an artificial, mechanical ventilator. The examining physician then reported to us that there was no apparent gas leakage into the skin, nothing in the neck or chest wall, but that his abdomen was becoming distended. Attempt at manual palpation of the abdomen revealed that it was almost as rigid as a board, indication that something catastrophic was happening in his abdominal cavity, producing signs of peritonitis, or an inflammation of the lining of the abdominal cavity. An X-ray revealed what appeared to be gas in the peritoneal cavity, probably the nitrogen produced from vaporization of the liquid nitrogen. The anesthesiologist, with the support of the toxicologist, was able to convince the surgeon to take the child to the operating room as an emergency with very little preparation prior to it for a presumption of a ruptured stomach. As things progressed, one could feel on physical examination, the presence of gas in his chest wall and in his neck. His abdomen was distended and it was felt that he was critically ill. His chest

X-ray revealed that there was free air below the diaphragm and there was no free air in the chest. A CAT scan of the chest and abdomen showed a large amount of air in the peritoneal cavity, the cavity around the organs in the stomach, and this led to his rapid movement to the operating room. Once in the operating room it was observed that there was widespread contamination of the peritoneal cavity. There was a ten centimeter (approximately four inches) perforation of the anterior (front) surface of the stomach adjacent to the lesser curvature. The surgeon stated that the young man's lunch was scattered throughout his peritoneal cavity, gastric contents and undigested food was seen "everywhere." The laceration was cleaned and repaired, the peritoneal cavity lavaged (washed out) with copious amounts of fluid to remove all remnants of the food that had escaped into it. A tube was surgically implanted into his intestines beyond the area of injury, so that he could receive feeding through the intestines,. If he had received nutrition only through his veins, the risk of infection would rise, so it was important to attempt to provide adequate calories and other nutrients through his normal intestines.

He underwent investigation of his esophagus and breathing pipe to be sure there were no injuries. There being none, the surgical site was closed and the patient left the operating room and was taken to the pediatric intensive care unit.

For the first three days of his postoperative hospital stay, he received no food by mouth, receiving nutrition solely by the intravenous route, and was kept on artificial ventilation. Postoperatively, he developed a shock syndrome and acute respiratory distress, and required support of his blood pressure and antibiotics, and was continued on a ventilator. On day four feeding was provided through the feeding tube, which had been placed into the small intestine at the time of the original surgery. This allowed feedings through his gastrointestinal tract, allowing better quality nutrition. On day eight, radiological evaluation showed no evidence of esophageal perforation or any obvious injury to or leakage at the surgical site in the stomach or small intestine. On day ten the endotracheal tube was removed and he was started on oral feedings after the endotracheal tube (breathing tube) was removed. He was then discharged from the pediatric intensive care unit, thirteen days after the initial surgery.

It was surprising to the staff at the poison center that we had not heard of this method of making ice cream before and so we searched the Internet and spoke to many high school and college students. It was determined that this procedure was widely known and both the demonstration and the use of this technique to make ice cream is done quite often.

Given the apparent widespread use of this technique, it was surprising to us that reported accidents related to it are not reported more often. We looked to see how easy it would be to purchase liquid nitrogen, whether it could be purchased without any license or credentials, and whether an adult would be required to purchase it. The staff of the poison center called several vendors in the counties surrounding the poison center, which had been found in a search of the yellow pages and on the Internet. We found several vendors willing to sell liquid nitrogen for the purpose of making ice cream. When the vendors were asked whether a teenager could purchase it for the class, without the presence of an adult, the vendor replied that as long as the teenager had the money to purchase the liquid nitrogen and provide a deposit fee for the canister needed to transport the liquid, they had no problem selling it to anyone without any identification or credentials. The vendors were more than willing to provide virtually any amount of liquid nitrogen that could be paid for by the consumer.

We discovered that the Internet is replete with recipes, descriptions, and even videos of the procedure. The fact that injury occurred was also somewhat shocking to us, as it appeared to us to demonstrate a total lack of control of this product. There is a lot to be learned from this case. Many years later, as I wrote this chapter, there are still no rules and or regulations concerning the sale, purchase, use, or storage of liquid nitrogen.

Suggested Reading

Berrizbeitia LD, Calello DP, Dhir N, et al. Liquid nitrogen ingestion followed by gastric perforation. Pediatr Emerg Care. 2010;26(1):1–3.

Pollard JS, Simpson JE. Gastric perforation after liquid nitrogen ingestion. Clin Toxicol. 2013;51(4):286–7.

Chapter 10
It Isn't Physiologically Possible!

There are many cities in the country that have lost their standing as commercially successful locations. The so called "rust belt," is replete with many towns and cities which were once prosperous and vital but which deteriorated into poverty and crime. Often such locations have evolved into hotbeds of drug abuse.

The call was received at midnight by Renato DeBellonia, one of the specialists at the poison center. An Emergency Department physician called about a strange case involving a twenty-five-year-old heroin abuser. The patient claimed that he believed that he had gotten a "bad batch" of heroin and that he was feeling "funny." The patient lived in one city, but bought his drugs "across the river" in another city, an almost mirror image demographically with the one in which he lived. Complicating matters later on, the two cities were in fact in different states. He stated that he purchased the heroin from his regular dealer in and snorted it as he usually did. He indicated that he regularly used heroin, snorting 2–3 times a week. There was nothing obviously different about this heroin or the circumstances until hours after he used it. He gave no indication of any other illness or previous medical problem. He did not think anyone was out to hurt him, or would want him dead. The emergency department reported that he came in hypotensive, with low blood pressure, and with a rapid heart rate and an elevated respiratory rate. One of the frequent causes of hypotension is an inadequate volume of circulating blood. The normal adult has about 5 L (each liter is a little greater than a quart) of blood in circulation. If the individual loses fluid by, for example, vomiting or diarrhea, he or she has a decrease in blood volume and this results in hypotension and usually a reflex increase in the heart rate. The circulatory system is not a static tube, its components, arteries and veins, are capable of constricting thus increasing blood flow rate and pressure, or dilating and producing hypotension and slow blood flow. In certain circumstances the circulatory system dilates to such a point as to create a virtual loss of blood through pooling in the circulatory system and the blood not returning properly to the heart. This is sometimes called "third spacing." The usual therapy offered is administering enough fluids, given intravenously, to fill the circulatory system and allow

© Springer International Publishing AG 2017
S.M. Marcus, *Medical Toxicology: Antidotes and Anecdotes*,
DOI 10.1007/978-3-319-51029-3_10

the contraction of the heart to move the blood around and resolve the hypotension. The patient was given intravenous fluids to try to bring his blood pressure up and received almost five liters of fluid (more than five quarts and about the average total blood volume in an adult) before his blood pressure rose and he started to produce urine, a good sign that his blood volume had been restored and his blood pressure was adequate enough to have his kidneys function correctly.

When the poison center was contacted we were told that his pupils were dilated, which would be strange since in most heroin overdoses the pupils are small, often described as pinpoint in size. A screen for toxins in his urine, also known as "urine tox" testing, was positive for opiates and benzodiazepines, not surprising since he admitted to using heroin which is an opiate. He was given benzodiazepine (in his case the emergency department used lorazepam, also known by its brand name Ativan) in the emergency department to try to calm him down because he was so agitated upon arrival. He was also found to test positive for marijuana, which in the drug-abusing population would not be unexpected.

His electrocardiogram showed a pattern suggesting "ischemic changes"—that is, his heart muscle was not receiving enough oxygen. This can occur when there is any obstruction or decrease in blood flow through the coronary arteries. The laboratory testing revealed a low potassium of 2.2 mmol/L. with the normal being 3.5–4.5, a low CO_2 of 19 mmol/L. with a normal range being of 25–35, and a glucose of 228 mg/dL which was more than double what you would expect it to be. There can be many causes of such abnormalities in laboratory testing and they were not immediately addressed in view of the need to address the other issues: agitation, hypotension, tachycardia, and possible cardiac muscle ischemia.

When dealing with an overdose, one frequently deals with a combination of physical findings and expressed symptoms that often suggest a specific poison. One of the first such combinations learned by students in all of the health fields, also called a toxidrome, is that for an opioid overdose. When one is presented with a patient showing altered mental status, depressed vital signs, and very small, "pinpoint" pupils, one considers the possibility of an opioid being involved; this is commonly called the opioid toxidrome. Unusual in this case was the fact that he had a rapid heartbeat and dilated pupils.

It was felt that the clinical effects were probably due to some contamination of the heroin, but what it consisted of was hard to know. Drug abusers often mix cocaine with their heroin forming what is known as a "speedball." The most famous victims of the effects of a speedball include John Belushi, Chris Farley, and Philip Seymour Hoffman, all of whom succumbed to an overdose of this combination. Cocaine produces an excitatory toxidrome usually consisting of agitation, tachycardia, hypertension, and dilated pupils. It is well documented that cocaine use can produce a chest-pain syndrome and this has been shown to relate to spasm of the coronary arteries and even obstruction of the coronary artery flow with resultant ischemic damage to the heart muscle. The possibility existed that the chest pain and abnormal cardiogram in this patient might have been evidence of cocaine-induced spasm of his coronary arteries. It was thought possible that the urine toxicology screen for cocaine was negative because of the way that test is done. A urine specimen obtained at a given time really represents what the kidneys produced since the last time the bladder was emptied. If a drug is used late in that time window, the drug might not be caught in a screen. The screen is sensitive to the concentration of a given drug in the urine. A negative test doesn't necessarily mean that there is no drug, but that its concentration is lower than that needed to produce a positive result. DeBellonia suggested the physician write orders to provide supportive care, intravenous fluids to increase his blood volume, and potassium to correct it to its normal range, as well as to watch the glucose and have cardiology take a look at the patient.

About four hours later the poison center received a call from another physician at the hospital stating that the patient became agitated and his heart rate rose to 140. The physician was so concerned that he ordered administration of medication to slow his heart down and calm him down. He was given diltiazem (Cardizem), a drug used both to lower blood pressure and to slow down the heart. It works by blocking the entry of calcium into cells, as calcium is the triggering ion which causes cells to contract. He was also given haloperidol (Haldol), a psychiatric drug used to calm patients that are agitated and distressed from psychiatric problems, primarily psychosis. Shortly after these medications were given, the patient's blood pressure dropped precipitously to the very low level of 60/13 mmHg. The hospital analyzed his blood and discovered that he had become acidemic, with a pH of 7.27 (normal being 7.35–7.45). He was breathing rapidly, producing a drop in the amount of carbon dioxide (CO_2) in his blood. His PCO_2—which is the measurement of the pressure of the gas CO_2 in the blood, normally in the range of 35–45—was below 30! This was odd, since when a person breathes fast, and as his PCO_2 drops, the individual usually becomes a bit alkalotic; that is, his or her pH rises, not lowers as this patient's did. There is a generally accepted "rule of thumb" that for every change in PCO_2 of 10 mmHg, there is a resultant drop in pH of 0.08 if the PCO_2 rises and a similar rise in pH if the PCO_2 drops, as we would have expected in this case. The fact that his pH did not rise above normal suggested that there was a derangement occurring in his metabolic pathway causing a metabolic acidosis. Generally, the human body has adequate buffers, substances that, even if there is a temporary derangement of metabolism, will help to correct the acidosis. The body has other homeostatic mechanisms to correct the acidosis, and the increase in respirations in response to the acidosis is generally the first line of defense. So it seemed obvious that the patient was suffering from a metabolic acidosis.

By this time we had the report of his blood work and he had what is called a wide anion gap. The human body consists of approximately 60% water that contains minerals and nutrients. These minerals are called electrolytes. The principle electrolytes measured in the body are sodium, potassium, chloride, and bicarbonate. These electrolytes carry electrical charges, hence the name electrolyte. There should be a balance between the positive charged and negative charged electrolytes. Sodium and potassium are the standard measured positive electrolytes, also called cations, while chloride and bicarbonate are the negatively charged ones, also called anions. When one compares the amount of positive and negative charged electrolytes as measured in the clinical laboratory, there is generally a small difference, with the negatively charged electrolytes, or anions, somewhat lower than the positively charged ones, or cations: the so-called anion gap. This is because there are other anions in the body that are generally not measured in the standard blood work. The normal anion gap, the difference between the total cations measured and that of the anions measured, should be less than twelve. This patient's anion gap was greater. There is a mnemonic that every medical student soon learns that helps in the differential diagnosis of a wide-anion-gap metabolic acidosis, A MUDPIE, also known as MUDPILES. Aspirin has many mechanisms, which combined produce a typical wide anion gap metabolic acidosis. Methanol or wood alcohol, can produce such an acidosis when it is converted by metabolism into its toxic metabolite, formic acid. In Diabetes mellitus (commonly just called diabetes), there is a potentially serious derangement which can occur, called diabetic keto-acidosis. In this situation, there is a lack of the proper amount of insulin to metabolize glucose for energy. The body is then forced to change from metabolizing glucose to the metabolism of fat to produce energy, termed lipolysis. Such lipolysis produces what are called keto-acids, beta-hydroxybutyric acid, and acetone, rapidly overwhelming the body's buffering system and producing the wide anion gap metabolic acidosis. Phenformin is an obsolete drug used in the treatment of diabetes, but its close relative, metformin, is commonly used. In patients overdosing on metformin, or diabetics who develop renal disease and take metformin, there may be a resultant wide anion gap metabolic acidosis. This acidosis is based on excess accumulation of lactic acid. The actual mechanism of induction of the metformin-associated metabolic acidosis is not clearly delineated, but is thought to be based on several mechanisms. The anti-tuberculosis drug Isoniazide, aka INH, is known to cause a wide anion gap metabolic acidosis, but most often only after the patient develops a seizure. INH interferes with the production of a substance in the brain to control excess activity, gamma amino butyric acid, aka GABA. Lack of this inhibitory substance leads to seizures and excess metabolism and a resultant wide anion gap metabolic acidosis. Some that like the mnemonic A MUDPIE consider the "I" also as a reminder of idiopathic lactic acidosis, more a result than a cause, but a useful reminder. Ethylene glycol, like methanol, has a metabolite which when existing in the blood will produce a wide anion gap metabolic acidosis. In the mnemonic MUDPILES, the L stands again for lactic acidosis and the S for salicylates, or aspirin. Debellonia started to think through the differential diagnosis, before calling the physicians and discussing his diagnoses with the treating physicians.

On his call back, he learned that the patient's pupils were still dilated and this was still troubling, since it was expected that the reverse would occur with an opioid in his system. Confusing to the treatment team was his lactic acid, which was elevated to 10.6 mmol/L, normally less than 4. Lactic acid becomes elevated when the body cannot metabolize sugar appropriately or when there is a large amount of muscular exertion. There also can be a false elevation in the laboratory analysis caused by a substance which interferes with the chemical identification of lactate. This can occur when antifreeze (usually consisting of ethylene glycol, remember the "E" in MUDPIES) is ingested, but there was no indication that he had been exposed to this.

Just after he hung up the phone with the original hospital, DeBellonia received a call about three other patients in another hospital, who were showing almost identical clinical features. This hospital was located in a different county far across the state. There was no commonality to the current case—no friendship, no geographical overlap—except for the commonality that the individuals were demonstrating almost the identical symptoms as the original, or index, patient or case.

When Debellonia reached out to me, I was startled by having patients in different hospitals who were demonstrating almost identical peculiar findings after exposure to heroin. Given the elevated lactic acid, persistent hypotension, and acidosis, the possibility of cyanide contamination of the heroin had to be raised. I suggested that a venous measurement of oxygen be determined and, if elevated, to go ahead and prophylactically treat all patents for cyanide poisoning.

Cyanide poisons the basic metabolic pathways throughout the body. The cytochrome system is the basis for almost all the metabolism that occurs in the body. Cyanide interferes with the exchange of electrons within the cytochrome system rendering the body incapable of utilizing oxygen by the tissues. This leads to the cells attempting to carry on their metabolic requirements through metabolism without the exchange of electrons normally donated by oxygen. This leads to the metabolic acidosis, and the elevation in lactate. Since there is no loss of oxygen from the arterial side of the blood circulation into the tissues, the oxygen in the venous side tends to be reported higher than normal. This is sometimes called "arterialization" of venous blood. The hospital did a venous PO_2 and found it was 76 mmHg (mercury). A venous PO_2 over 50 mmHg is very unusual. Even in individuals inhaling 100% oxygen, the tissues are so efficient at removing oxygen that it is unlikely that the PO_2 will ever rise above 50 mmHg. Informed of this, my suggestion was to start the patient on one of the cyanide antidotes available at that time, sodium thiosulfate. Sodium thiosulfate is capable of reacting with cyanide and produces thiocyanate, which can be cleared from the body by the kidneys excreting the substance in the urine. Approximately an hour later the hospital called back and said the patient was feeling better after having received the thiosulfate, and his blood pressure was now normal and his heart rate had slowed a bit. That suggested that the offending agent might indeed be cyanide, but was there cyanide in the heroin and if so why?

After another hour the patient began breathing rapidly again and appeared anxious. He was asking for "Valium," the brand name for the benzodiazepine diazepam. The hospital repeated his venous PO_2 and it was now over 100 mmHg. He was given another dose of sodium thiosulfate. Again he transiently improved and became less anxious while his breathing slowed down. He subsequently developed extreme agitation and the treating team was forced to administer a drug similar to diazepam (Valium), lorazepam. This medication was ordered to be given intravenously, around the clock.

The patient began complaining that his head was hurting and he was found to have a heart rate of 135 and a respiratory rate of twenty seven, his blood pressure dropped to 79/40 mmHg. By now we had used so much thiosulfate that the hospital was running out of its supply. We reached out to the state health department to locate additional supplies of sodium thiosulfate. In addition we reported to the state health department that we now had a total of nine patients, three patients each, in three different hospitals in three different counties of the state all with the same picture, and that we were concerned that this might be a possible terrorist action defined as someone contaminating heroin. All nine patients presented within twelve hours of each other. We reached out to the local agencies in the involved communities, the Pennsylvania State Police, the New Jersey State Police, and the Philadelphia and the New York City Poison Centers to alert them of the events that had been transpiring. In addition we contacted the county prosecutors' offices for the counties in which the nine victims were being treated.

I received a telephone call from the New Jersey Commissioner of Health requesting information on what was transpiring. I explained that we had an outbreak involving nine patients, three in each of three counties, and that physiologically it appeared that they were all suffering from a toxin, as was considering that it could be cyanide, that was causing the arterialization of venous blood. I stated that I had "one foot out the door" to drive to the hospital to see if I could shine any light on what was going on. The commissioner's comment to me was, "Do you know how far the hospital is?" My response was "I really don't know, and really don't care. There are sick patients and they need me. I will be there at the bedside to do whatever I can." I then got into my car and drove to the hospital of the initial patients, a trip of a little over an hour from my home.

There are two antidotes for cyanide poisoning. The classic approach is the administration of a drug, sodium nitrite, which induces methemoglobinemia, an oxidized form of hemoglobin. Cyanide although binding tightly to hemoglobin, does not bind well to methemoglobin; in fact, it is thought that one can "detach" cyanide from hemoglobin by converting that hemoglobin into methemoglobin. The problem with this approach is that nitrites produce dilatation of the blood vessels and hypotension, or shock. Our patient was already suffering from a low blood pressure, so that was not considered a viable option. Once cyanide is released from the hemoglobin it is bound to the administered thiosulfate and, as discussed earlier, is cleared from the body by the kidneys. There is a new antidote, cobalamin, which can be used and does not produce the hypotension that is seen with nitrite administration. When cobalamin is administered, it combines with the cyanide and produces the substance cyanocobalamine, also known as vitamin B12. Its major side effects are the reddish discoloration of the recipient's tissues and secretions and the color interferes with some laboratory tests which are based on colorimetric assays. The antidote has been reported to increase blood pressure in volunteers receiving the drug. Whereas this side effect might be a nuisance in a volunteer, in a real victim who is hypotensive this rise in blood pressure, if it is due to the drug, might be advantageous in the clinical theatre. It would have been a great time to use the antidote, however it was not yet widely available in the United States, and none of the hospitals in which the patients were hospitalized nor any hospital close by stocked this new, more expensive medication. There is evidence that thiosulfate by binding with the cyanide in circulation and then being excreted in the urine, can move the equilibrium of cyanide binding and cause the elimination of cyanide and improvement in the victim. This is what we believed we were experiencing with our patients at that time.

Upon arrival I saw a well-developed young man who was in no distress. He had a heart rate of 112 beats per minute and a respiratory rate of 22 breaths per minute. By that time he had received seven doses of sodium thiosulfate and one dose of sodium nitrite in an attempt to treat what we believed was cyanide contamination of heroin.

I was an eyewitness to a nurse drawing blood from the patient's vein and remarked that the redness of the blood certainly looked as if it was arterial and asked her whether she was sure that she had drawn from a vein and not an artery. To prove to myself that the blood was truly venous, I drew a sample myself and in fact his venous blood was bright red (see Fig. 10.1). Considering the overall clinical picture, we made the decision to induce methemoglobinemia by administering sodium nitrite. He seemed, once again, to improve from our treatment. His methemoglobin level rose to 6.8% and his symptoms "disappeared."

Before I left the hospital the patient seemed to be improving, as he was calm and was no longer complaining of a headache or any discomfort. Unfortunately, his repeat methemoglobin level had dropped. Since he was by now asymptomatic, we elected not to give him more correction. When I reached home and spoke to the hospital treatment team, I learned that his methemoglobin level had dropped to 1.8% and his venous PO_2 rose to 181 mmHg. I suggested giving him another dose of sodium nitrite and to repeat the methemoglobin level and venous blood gases after that. Later that afternoon, one day after admission, the patient was very weak but was relieved that he was doing better. His methemoglobin level was now 6.1 but his venous PO_2 was still 115 mmHg. He received another dose of sodium nitrite and yet another dose of sodium thiosulfate. His vital signs revealed a blood pressure of 105/50 mmHg, heart rate of 100, and respiratory rate 20s.

Fig. 10.1 The center vial is a control sample, actually my own blood, which appears darker than the other two tubes of blood flanking it which were bright red and came from two victims' veins

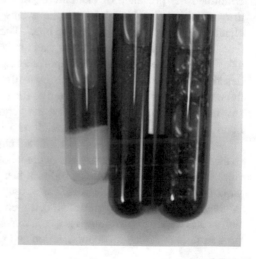

That evening I consulted by telephone with the treating doctors; his venous PO_2 dropped to 59 mmHg, his methemoglobin was 3.2% and the patient was asymptomatic. The following day his venous PO_2 rose again to over 200 mmHg, his methemoglobin was 3.8%, and he was developing some symptoms suggestive of heroin withdrawal so we suggested that he be started on methadone. On the morning of the third hospital day his venous PO_2 was 162 mmHg rising to 191 mmHg, and he continued to receive sodium thiosulfate.

Summarizing the situation in my mind, there were three hospitals with three patients in each, all with similar histories and clinical effects. All three patients at the first hospital were seen by me and were being monitored closely with blood gas and methemoglobin determinations. All three had elevated venous PO_2s and were, by this time, asymptomatic. Not really knowing what we were dealing with, I brought a sample of blood from each of the three patients into the Regional Medical Examiner's Office located near my office in Newark, New Jersey. The medical examiner's laboratory performed a rapid qualitative test for cyanide, which revealed no presence.

The combination of the lack of confirmation of cyanide and the fact that the patients were relatively asymptomatic at that point, despite having elevations of venous PO_2, led us to suggest stopping the therapy. On the fifth hospital day we were able to locate a bag of "leftover" heroin that one of the patients was willing to give us. I obtained that specimen and provided some to both the Pennsylvania and the New Jersey State Police for evaluation.

Within a short time after the drug was received by the state police laboratory, we were contacted by the technician and told that there was *no heroin* found in the sample. The technician charged with the responsibility of analyzing the specimen was usually involved in testing of thoroughbred horses that raced in the state to ensure that there was no "doping" or performance enhancing drugs given to those horses. One look at the output curve from the analyzer and the technologist "knew" that it was not heroin, and that it was the banned substance clenbuterol. The FBI lab confirmed the presence of clenbuterol, quinine, and mannitol in the specimen of drug collected. Looking back on the events and the data we collected, we were clearly led astray by our "anchoring bias." There is the tale of eight blind men, blind from birth, who had never seen or had an experience with an elephant. On being asked to describe what they felt upon feeling the trunk of the elephant, each man described it in relationship to their own life experiences, all totally different and none were correct. When we were presented with the situation as it unfolded, we saw only the clinical symptoms and the venous arterializations and the history of heroin exposure, we did not pay attention to the low potassium and high blood sugars with co-existing rapid heart rate, dilated pupils, and agitation. We were "blinded" to the fact that all of these are signs of catecholamine excess. The hormone epinephrine, also known as adrenalin, produces just this effect. These catecholamines all work by stimulating the Na-K ATPase pump. That pump is responsible for maintaining the normal charge across all cell membranes in the body (the resting potential, as it is called in physiology), which makes the cell slightly polarized and ready for a stimulus to force its depolarization and producing whatever activity that cell is "programmed" to perform. The pump pushes potassium into the cell and pumps sodium out. When an impulse from a nerve hits the cell membrane, which is charged and ready to go, the pump ceases and potassium leaves the cell while sodium and its companion calcium enter the cell. This change ends up producing whatever the specific cell is programmed to do. If a muscle cell, it is then stimulated to contract, if the cell is programmed to produce and then release (e.g., insulin), then insulin will be released. Excessive stimulation of the pump, for example, by administering a medication like clenbuterol, will push additional potassium into the cell. This can be used for clinical advantage. Such an increase in the pumping of potassium into the cells makes the cell more polarized and thus more difficult to get it depolarized and therefore react. If that cell happens to be one of the muscle cells surrounding the airway and the airway is constricted, adding a medication that causes the pump to work "overtime" may cause the muscle to go into its resting, or relaxed, state, thus producing dilatation of the airway. Clenbuterol happens to be one drug that does stimulate that effect, and can be used for asthma to relax the airway. One of the other effects of such catecholamines is the stimulation of the breakdown of the glycogen that is stored in the liver in a process called glycogenolysis, which produces an increase in glucose. Thus, it should have come as no surprise that the victims of the use of this drug became hypokalemic (had low potassium) and hyperglycemic (had increased blood glucose).

There are two main receptors involved in the catecholamine system. In cell biology, a receptor is a structure on the surface of a cell (or inside a cell) that selectively receives and binds a specific substance. The two main catecholamine receptors are the alpha and beta receptors. Stimulation of these receptors is what produces the demonstrable effects of the catecholamine system. The alpha receptors are mostly in the arterial walls, and stimulation produces constriction and increase in blood pressure. The beta receptor has two subtypes: one, the beta$_1$ receptor, is in cardiac (heart) tissue and stimulation produces both an increase in force of contraction (so called inotropy) and speeds up the heart rate (so called chronotropy). The other receptor, the beta$_2$, tends to be more of a smooth muscle relaxer, causing relaxation in the muscles surrounding the walls of arteries and producing vasodilatation upon stimulation, and dilatation of the muscles surrounding respiratory tissues causing a widening of the tracheo-bronchial tree. This renders beta agonist therapy of prime importance when treating patients with broncho-constriction, as in cases of asthma.

Clenbuterol has an interesting effect on the growth of muscle mass. Animals given the drug have dramatic increases in their muscle mass. Research has shown that this occurs without the release of insulin or any other hormone. Sometimes incorrectly called an anabolic steroid, clenbuterol does not seem to exhibit such effects in man, and the increase in muscle mass produced in man is not yet explained.

Soon after the substance was identified, there was a telephone conference between the New Jersey Department of Health, the New Jersey State Police, and the poison center on what to do with the information about this "contaminated" and dangerous drug. There was a great deal of argument about what to call it since it was purchased as heroin but actually had no heroin in it. There was belief that we should not be calling it contaminated heroin but this led to the difficulty of how we might describe the situation to the press or to those who might be at risk for exposure. The state police decided that we should not waste time and sent out the word that there was dangerous contaminated heroin on the streets. Public health did not like this approach because its belief was that all illicit drugs are dangerous and therefore it would be difficult to tell people that this particular batch was dangerous.

I posted an alert about the drug on the United States Centers for Disease Control's epidemic alert network, Epi-X. This network was established sometime after the post 9/11 anthrax scare to link epidemiologists and other important health officials into a secure network that could send out blast alerts to everyone who subscribed to the network. As a medical director of a regional poison center, I had such access. I described the situation and developed a case definition so that epidemiologists all across the country would be on the lookout and report any exposures that they became aware of in their communities. The working case definition included individuals who used heroin and developed acidosis, hypotension, hypokalemia, and elevated glucose and, as an aside, elevated venous PO_2. The alert went through Epi-X to all poison center directors who were subscribers. To wear both suspenders and a belt, I also sent an alert through regular email to all medical and managing directors of poison centers. Shortly thereafter cases began to appear in New York, Connecticut, and North Carolina. Before the outbreak seemed to "burn" itself out, there were cases reported all along the eastern coastline of the United States.

To my knowledge, there was no further investigation; as to the source of the substance, the perpetrators of its sale have never been found. Public health officials told me that since drug abuse is illegal, this was not a public health matter.

Postscript

Clenbuterol was a popular but banned drug used by athletes in bodybuilding, power-related activities, and even in endurance sports. Purchased through the Internet, it is commonly used by body builders for "fat burning" and to increase muscle mass. "Cheating" with clenbuterol has been seen at 4-H shows in an attempt to bulk up animals. Outbreaks of poisoning in people that ate meat from animals fed clenbuterol have been reported. In Spain and Portugal, over 100 people developed nervousness, rapid heart rate, muscle shaking, muscle pain, and headache fifteen minutes to six hours after eating veal liver.[1,2] These symptoms lasted from ninety minutes to six days. Testing of those individuals showed very low blood levels of clenbuterol but very high levels of urinary clenbuterol, suggesting that the drug is eliminated and concentrated in the urine. Poison centers still receive isolated calls

[1] Salleras L, Dominguez A, Mata E, et al. (1995) Epidemiologic study of an outbreak of clenbuterol poisoning in Catatonia, Spain. Public Health Reports 110(3):338–342.

[2] Barbosa J, Cruz C, Martins J, et al. (2005) Food poisoning by clenbuterol in Portugal. Food Additives Contamination. 22(6):563–566.

in which the patient has symptoms and signs consistent with case definition. No one has ever disclosed why the drug has been used to replace heroin, and no person responsible for the substitution has ever been found.

Suggested Reading

Hoffman RS, Kirrane B, Marcus SM. A descriptive study of an outbreak of clenbuterol-containing heroin. Ann Emerg Med. 2008;52(5):548–53.

Hoffman RS, Nelson LS, Chan GM, et al. A typical reactions associated with heroin use-five states, January-April 2005. MMWR. 2005;54(32):793–6.

Chapter 11
Color Me Red

I was at my desk one morning when the phone rang. It was my staff assistant telling me that there was a pediatrician on the phone who was asking questions about lead poisoning. The call was from a pediatrician calling about a patient. Dr. Patel (pseudonym) had been a pediatric resident I worked with when I was an assistant director of pediatrics. She was calling about a child she just discovered had lead poisoning, and was asking for advice. She had not encountered a child with lead poisoning in many years and needed some input from me.

As lead builds up in a child's body, it poisons many vital bodily functions. There are so many enzyme systems poisoned by lead that there is virtually no organ system that is not at risk from the effects of lead. One of the most important systems to be poisoned is the synthesis of heme. Heme is the pigment which is part of the hemoglobin in the red cells of the body and gives the cells their characteristic red color. Hemoglobin is responsible for transporting vital oxygen through the body. Heme is also involved with metabolism (for example, of sugar) throughout the body to produce energy for the body. Within the mitochondria of all cells, the amino acid glycine reacts with succinyl-COA, from the Kreb's cycle, to produce the intermediary compound D-aminolevulinic acid (dALA or δALA). This substance then leaves the mitochondria and is dehydrogenated by the enzyme d-aminolevulenic acid dehydrogenase (dALAD) to porphobilinogen, the first of the porphyrins to be produced in the synthetic pathway. This is an important step because the enzyme involved, dALAD, is exquisitely sensitive to lead. With lead exposure there may be such a severe block at this stage that the entire pathway is blocked, leading to decreased heme production and resulting in anemia. The synthetic pathway then continues in the cytoplasm with the sequential production of porphobilinogen, hydroxymethyl bilane, uroporphyrinogen, and then coproporphyrinogen, which then diffuses back into the mitochondiran and becomes protoporphyrinogen III and then protoporphyrin IX. Iron then diffuses into the mitochondria and is complexed with protoporphyrin IX by the enzyme ferrochelatase and becomes heme. The heme then diffuses out of the mitochondrion and binds to the protein globin, producing hemoglobin. This later enzyme, ferrochelatase, is sensitive to the effects of lead,

© Springer International Publishing AG 2017
S.M. Marcus, *Medical Toxicology: Antidotes and Anecdotes*,
DOI 10.1007/978-3-319-51029-3_11

which causes a block in the synthesis of heme and thus decreased hemoglobin (and anemia) and a buildup of protoporphyrin IX. Heme is an essential component of other substances as well as hemoglobin. Oxidative phosphorylation is the term used to describe the principal ways that organisms produce energy. Essential to this process is the presence of cytochromes, hemeproteins. The basic "factory" producing energy resides in the mitochondria. These cytochromes, by the process of oxidation and reduction, produce adenosine triphosphate, ATP, the universal chemical "currency" of energy needed for all vital functions of every organism. Lead in its interference with heme synthesis, interferes with the function of these cytochromes, producing widespread effects throughout the organism.

New Jersey had a large percentage of wood-frame homes which were built prior to the 1950s and were painted with lead based paint. As the paint deteriorated, it chipped off of the walls, ceilings, and woodwork and fell to the floor, where crawling children would ingest the chips and develop lead poisoning. In 1972, when I first moved my clinical work to New Jersey, almost 50% of the children we screened for lead were found to have elevated lead levels high enough to be said to have "lead poisoning." Lead poisoning is most dangerous for its neurological implications. Children can develop seizures or fall into a comatose state. Less severe can be hyperactivity, irritability, or loss of recently acquired skills. Even if children remain asymptomatic, they may later develop learning disabilities or other complications.

Because of the number of children diagnosed with lead poisoning between 1970 and 2000, my hospital's pediatric department ran three "lead clinics" a week. We saw between 15 and 20 children during each clinic. There was nearly always a child in the hospital being treated for lead poisoning. With federal laws enacted banning the use of lead-based paint and massive public health and environmental intervention by the start of the twenty-first century that figure dropped to below 10%.

During Dr. Patel's residency, lead poisoning was a common diagnosis. She learned how to be alert to the problem. Following the suggestions of the American Academy of Pediatrics and the required regulations of the New Jersey Department of Health and Senior Services, the doctor screened an approximately one-year-old girl for lead. To the doctor's surprise the lead level was reported at 57 mcg/dL. At that point the United States Centers for Disease Control and Prevention considered an elevation in blood lead level over 25 mcg/dL as significant. Most of us considered a lead level of 57 mcg/dL as an emergency, one that could produce an acute, serious problem such as convulsions or coma. My reaction to Dr. Patel's was surprise that despite the fact that the child lived in a low-risk area, the child was found to have such an elevation in blood lead level. Dr. Patel was in a mild state of panic trying to determine what to do with the child.

The treatment of childhood lead poisoning is primarily to separate the child from the source of lead and thus my suggestion was to have the child admitted to the hospital so that we might protect the child from any further exposure. We would then evaluate the environmental situation and find the source of exposure to lead and eliminate it. At the same time we would administer medication to the child in order to decrease her blood lead level, so-called chelation therapy. Dr. Patel thanked me for my help and agreed to admit the child to the hospital. Not long after that discussion, the father called the poison center and spoke to one of our information specialists concerned that the child would be admitted to an appropriate institution and treated correctly. He also asked if we knew if a lead level could be done on a Sunday. He questioned whether the blood test was accurate. The specialist explained to the father that if that blood test was done in the regular routine lab then it could be trusted and that, although Sunday is other people's day off, most clinical laboratories operate on Saturdays and Sundays and holidays as well. The father thanked the specialist and said yes that they would follow up and admit the child to the hospital.

The child was admitted. There was some confusion at the hospital concerning a repeat level of lead done at the hospital. The hospital had purchased a lead analysis machine, a "point-of-service" device to measure blood lead levels. When tested on their machine, the child's blood lead level was reported to be only 28 mcg/dL, a fraction of the outpatient result obtained from an outside reference laboratory by the child's pediatrician. The hospital's utilization people wanted the child discharged immediately. Not trusting the hospital's machine, since it was not designed for use as a reference instrument in a hospital, we had a sample of blood done at the laboratory at the New Jersey Medical School at the University of Medicine and Dentistry of New Jersey (now known as the New Jersey Medical School of the School of Biomedical and Health Sciences of Rutgers University). That laboratory confirmed the original blood level that was done in an outside reference laboratory. This opened up a series of discussions with the manufacturer of the hospital's point-of-service lead analyzer. That issue was eventually resolved by the equipment manufacturer with a recall of the reagents used in the measurement and, eventually, a redesign of the machine itself.

The most important part of treatment of lead poisoning is to look for and remove any source of lead. The local health department was contacted and asked to do a home inspection. Within twenty-four hours, the local health department conducted a home inspection and interviewed the family. They reported back that they couldn't find a source of lead exposure and felt the family history revealed no indication of risk. Confusing as well was the fact that an abdominal X-ray taken of the child in the hospital revealed no evidence of recently ingested substances that might contain lead. There was serious question as to what was going on, what was causing the child to have such an elevated blood lead level.

Further history revealed that the baby was mostly breast-fed but it was also eating some food prepared by the parents. Dr. Patel asked that we test the mother's breast milk to determine whether the child's exposure occurred from exposure to breast milk. She theorized that the mother became lead poisoned while she was growing up in her native India and had a large lead body burden and was then giving that lead to her child through her breast milk. It is known that once ingested, lead becomes distributed in several areas of the body. It demonstrates what is known as a multi-compartment model. There is some lead in the blood but that represents very little of the total body burden of lead. The blood is then in equilibrium with the soft tissues or organs of the body, such as the heart, liver, kidneys, and brain. Those are in turn in equilibrium with the boney tissues. These equilibriums allow the movement of lead in both directions but favors the movement of lead from the blood to soft tissues and then bone. The bones of the body function as ultimate storage sites. The estimated half-life of lead in bone, that is the time in which half of the lead in bone will leach out into the tissues, is about ten years. Thus an exposure in childhood may very well remain in the bones into the child-bearing years. It has been shown in lower animals that the movement from the bone back into the soft tissues and blood is facilitated by both pregnancy and breast feeding. So the possibility of such breast milk contamination had to be considered. Although at that time we did have the capability of doing breast-milk analysis, we felt that it would be far better to determine what the mother's blood lead level was rather than her breast milk. If the mother's blood lead was not elevated, it would be highly unlikely that the breast milk would be elevated, and it's far easier to do a blood lead level test. A sample of blood was obtained from the mother and transported to us at the poison center and was analyzed, as an emergency, at the laboratory in the Department of Preventive Medicine and Community Health at the New Jersey Medical School of the University of Medicine and Dentistry of New Jersey. The mother's blood lead level revealed a result of 85 mcg/dL, a startling result considering that the mother had no known risk factors for exposure. She had grown up in India but did not work in any occupation that would put her at risk and had no other risk factors. The mother denied having a habit of putting things into her mouth or eating nonfood substances, a habit called pica. Because the mother and the child had elevated blood lead levels, the physician tested the father and found that his blood lead level was, amazingly, 95 mcg/dL. The existence of elevated blood lead levels in all three members of the family strongly indicated a common exposure. It intensified the need to find the source of the lead exposure and eliminate it.

Meanwhile in the hospital, post chelation, the child's lead level dropped to 22 mcg/dL and the hospital wished to have the child discharged, but lacking an obvious source of exposure and thus obviously unable to eliminate the chance of re-exposure, we were reluctant to do so.

With all the family members demonstrating elevated blood lead levels it was felt that there had to be a common source of lead somewhere in the home. The health department was asked to reinvestigate for any possible source of lead in the home environment. After another visit to the home, the inspector from the health department reported, once again, that there was no source of lead in their home.

So the conundrum continued. It was clear that the family was being exposed to lead and that there appeared to be a common source of exposure to lead but the health department had been unable to find a source. Since all of the family members continued to reveal elevations in blood lead levels, a licensed lead inspector from the local health department, accompanied by the epidemiologist from the poison center, went back to visit the family in their home. They were told by me to not leave anything untested, to open every cabinet, inspect every item of food, food preparation—in fact, everything the family had in the house until they found the source. In discussion with the family, there was no obvious occupational exposure which could have resulted in "fouling of the nest." The mother was a full-time, stay-at-home mother. The father was working but his job did not involve contact with lead or any known lead products. Neither parent had any hobby which might expose the family to lead. The main focus of the investigation then turned to the fact that the family was of South Asian, non-Hindu origin and used a variety of ethnic food products as food additives. During the visit samples were collected of the more than 15 different remedies, spices, and cooking products found in the house and, in addition, a sample of breast milk was collected.

A day later an additional visit was made to the family's home. Again the lead inspector and the epidemiologist returned, but this time they brought a portable X-ray fluorescence analyzer, an XRF lead detection device. This device uses a radioactive source that, when applied to a lead containing substance, reads out in parts of lead found per million. It was used to test toys, cooking utensils, and other substances and objects in the home. This device identified two items that raised concern as possible sources of lead exposure. One of these items was a frying pan which showed lead on its exterior surface, the second item was a small container labeled "Sindoor, product of India, not edible." The mother was asked what the sindoor was used for, and she stated that she been used it as a food coloring over the preceding several weeks. She claimed that she had purchased this at a local grocery store as it was displayed near the check out counter. She asked the clerk at the checkout counter if it could be used as a food coloring and was told that, "only as long as a little bit is used." The family used the substance as a food dye to color their chicken red-orange.

The container of sindoor and the frying pan, along with other samples collected, were taken to the laboratory of the Department of Preventive Medicine and Community Health at the University of Medicine and Dentistry's New Jersey Medical School for further analysis. The materials were analyzed for their lead concentration. Dr. John Bogden, who supervised the laboratory, confirmed that the sindoor had the highest lead content among the collected samples and was 58% lead by weight. He stated that the breast milk contained tiny concentrations of lead but more than would normally be expected. Additionally, the frying pan had a significant amount of lead on the surface as determined by wiping it and then analyzing the wipes. The results suggested that long-term consumption of the breast milk and of the food prepared in the frying pan could certainly contribute to the high blood lead levels in the family. The family was visited and cautioned about the use of sindoor and the family was instructed to cease using anything except approved food dyes and substances manufactured by reputable companies in food preparation. A press release was issued to alert health professionals and local communities about the risk of lead poisoning from sindoor.

A survey of five randomly selected South Asian grocery stores was performed to see if there was sindoor sold in the stores. At each store an employee was asked if they ever sold sindoor and what was the common use. They were further asked if it could be used as a food coloring. Two of the stores were out of stock, and two stores had sindoor. In two stores, sindoor was sold in tightly sealed plastic containers. The outer label of the containers clearly stated the name of the product and the warning "nonedible." The fifth store had sindoor but it was in an unlabeled plastic bag, such as what the family stated that they saw in the grocery store. These bags did not display the name of the product nor a warning label. It was a general consensus among the surveyed employees of all five stores that sindoor is meant to be used only for cosmetic and religious purposes and should not be added to food. Investigation by local health officials found a restaurant using sindoor as a dye for its tandoori chicken. The restaurant was issued a fine, closed, and ordered decontaminated before being allowed to re-open with the understanding that it would cease using any non-approved food ingredients.

Sindoor, also called vermilion, is a pigment used as a "cosmetic" in the Hindu culture. It is used, traditionally, either as the forehead dot, or bindi, or in the part of the hair in married women, or maang. A similar preparation kumkuma is also available. There is another product kajal, also known as kohl, which has been traditionally used as eye makeup, similarly to the use of mascara. This preparation has also been reported as containing high levels of lead and has been related to the occurrence of elevated blood lead levels in small children whose parents apply the substance to their eyes.[1]

Back to our patient: after we found the source of lead exposure and chelated the child, allowing her blood level to drop, she was discharged from the hospital. Followed by her pediatrician, her blood lead level dropped to an acceptable range and never rose again.

Soon after the discovery of the family with lead poisoning from sindoor and the publication of the warnings, we heard of other outbreaks similar to this that occurred in other areas of the United States as well as in India itself.

Postscript

In 2015 a candidate for his Ph.D. at the Rutgers University School of Public Health, in the course of conducting his thesis, surveyed both local stores and the Internet and purchased samples of sindoor and kumkuma. Analysis of this substance, which he bought as intended to be used as a cosmetic, contained lead in as high as 98%, also known as 980,000 ppm. This far exceeds the United States Food and Drug Administration (FDA) standard of 20 ppm, or 0.0020%.[2] He also determined that a significant amount of the sindoor was "imported" by the individual women or their families from India when they immigrated to the United States or returned from a visit to their homeland.

In the spring of 2016, a family living in an older city in New Jersey, concerned about the possible exposure to lead in drinking water had their toddler tested for lead. The results showed a blood lead level of 30 mcg/dL in the child and 15 mcg/dL in the mother. Inspection of the home revealed no lead in the construction but the mother had been using kumkuma. In addition she was using a medication she

[1] Mohta A. Kajal (Kohl)—A dangerous cosmetic (2010) Oman J Ophthalmol. 3(2):100–101.
[2] FDA Lead in Cosmetics. http://www.fda.gov/Cosmetics/ProductsIngredients/PotentialContaminants/ucm388820.htm accessed 27 March 2016.

imported from India, an ayurvedic preparation. Such preparations have long been known to contain lead.[3] Analysis of the kumkuma and the ayurvedic mediations revealed significant levels of lead, well above the danger point.

Since the international airports in New Jersey, New York, and Massachusetts are major ports of arrival from India into the United States and since many newly arriving individuals would likely be carrying sindoor, kohl, ayurvedic medications, or similar lead-containing products, we requested that a warning sign or signs be placed in the waiting area for immigration/passport control. Unfortunately, as of August 2016, this had not occurred.

Suggested Reading

FDA warns consumers not to use Swad brand sindoor: product contains high levels of lead. FDA News Release, December 15, 2007. http://www.fda.gov/NewsEvents/Newsroom/PressAnnouncements/2007/ucm109040.htm.

Lin CG, Scheider LA, Brabander DJ, et al. Pediatric lead exposure from imported Indian spices and cultural powders. Pediatrics. 2010;125(4):e828–35.

Vassilev ZP, Marcus SM, Ayyanathan K, et al. Case of elevated blood lead in a South Asian family that has used Sindoor for food coloring. Clin Toxicol. 2005;43:301–3.

---

[3] Araujo J, AP Beelen AP, Lewis LD. Lead Poisoning Associated with Ayurvedic Medications— Five States, 2000–2003. MMWR (2004) 53(26): 582–584.

Chapter 12
My Baby Won't Eat

It was just after lunch on a beautiful spring day, when a poison information specialist at the New Jersey Poison Center, and Bruce Ruck, the managing director, appeared at my office. They wanted to discuss a very interesting case and asked me to speak to a pediatric resident from a teaching hospital about an infant in their pediatric intensive care unit. The resident had called asking about how to treat a baby with the "gasping syndrome."

In 1981 sixteen neonatal deaths were described with such a syndrome. Detective work by the pediatricians involved reported that the syndrome was associated with the use of benzyl alcohol preservative in some intravascular solutions (IVs) and were reported to the United States Food and Drug Administration (FDA) by two medical centers. The deaths occurred in pre-term neonates who had intravenous catheters flushed periodically with bacteriostatic (designed to prevent infection) normal saline solutions containing benzyl alcohol. The reported onset of toxicity in the infants occurred between several days and a few weeks of age with a characteristic clinical picture that included metabolic acidosis (the presence of excess acid in their blood) resulting in what appeared to be respiratory distress and "gasping" respirations. Many infants developed convulsions and hypotension (low blood pressure) leading to cardiovascular collapse and death.

The "gasping syndrome" was subsequently characterized as belonging to a child exposed to benzoyl alcohol, with hypotension, bradycardia, gasping respiration, hypotonia, progressive metabolic acidosis, seizures, cardiovascular collapse, and death.

Benzyl alcohol is an aromatic alcohol usually used in a concentration of 0.9% as a bacteriostatic preservative in multiple-dose vials of solutions or drugs for parenteral therapy. It is normally oxidized rapidly to benzoic acid, conjugated with glycine in the liver, and excreted as hippuric acid. Toxicological analysis of the neonates, suffering from the gasping syndrome, revealed benzyl alcohol or its metabolites in blood and urine samples from infants. Further analysis of urine samples from infants showed benzoate and hippurate, metabolites of benzoyl alcohol.

© Springer International Publishing AG 2017
S.M. Marcus, *Medical Toxicology: Antidotes and Anecdotes*,
DOI 10.1007/978-3-319-51029-3_12

Based on these reports, the FDA recommended that intravascular flush solutions containing benzyl alcohol not be used for newborns and that diluents with this preservative not be used as medications for these infants.

Dr. Ruck and the specialist said they had spoken to the resident from a hospital's pediatric intensive care unit. She was questioning the specialist about the treatment for sodium benzoate poisoning. The resident related the fact that she was caring for a three-month-old female who had been admitted to the hospital six days previously for sepsis, an infection of her bloodstream. The infant was being treated with antibiotics but was not getting any better. When the resident spoke to the mother she discovered that the baby had not been feeding well for several days and seemed to be gassy, and she had purchased an over-the-counter medication which was supposed to help with gastrointestinal problems. When the baby started developing what the resident described as "gasping respirations," the resident remembered learning about the gasping syndrome and its association with benzoyl alcohol. She looked up the medication and found that it contained sodium benzoate as a preservative. The resident having just rotated through the neonatal intensive care unit, had learned about the gasping syndrome and thought that perhaps this was what the baby was suffering from, due to the benzoate, and wanted direction as to what to do to help the child. My experience told me that sodium benzoate is a salt that would not metabolize or convert back to any of the putative causes of gasping syndrome. I wanted to learn more about the infant and her course of illness, because I believed that the diagnosis of sepsis was incorrect and that the child might be suffering from infant botulism.

Infant botulism is the most common botulinum syndrome reported in the United States. There are approximately 100 reported cases each year. The typical case occurs when an infant under six months of age (the median age being three months) is breast fed and presents with a sepsis-like clinical picture consisting of lethargy, poor sucking and crying, and decreased or absent stooling. Dr. Stephen Arnon, a pediatrician in California, was responsible for defining the diagnosis and reporting it in the medical literature in 1976 and developed the antidote, which is available through the California Department of Health. The antidote must be started as quickly as possible to avoid progression of the illness to the point at which an infant needs to have a breathing tube inserted and be placed on a mechanical ventilator. I knew that with six days already behind us, and the baby appearing to be deteriorating, the clock was ticking faster and faster towards such a situation. I needed to speak to the resident, confirm my belief through further history, and get the hospital mobilized to obtain the antidote.

The specialist set up a conference call for me to speak to the resident. I introduced myself and congratulated her for "thinking outside of the box," and for calling for our advice. I explained about sodium benzoate and the fact that as a salt, it was not convertible back to benzoyl alcohol or any of its toxic metabolites. I then went into greater depth with the resident about the history.

The resident recounted the history: this was the first child born to a twenty-six-year-old mother, the result of an uncomplicated first pregnancy. The baby was born vaginally, with a weight of eight pounds. She was breast fed with formula supplementation and was discharged with her mother. When the baby was one week of age, the mother ran out of the supplemental formula supplied by the hospital and went to a Woman and Infant Clinics (WIC) clinic. These federally funded clinics— officially the Special Supplemental Nutrition Program for Women, Infants, and Children (WIC)—provide "Federal grants to States for supplemental foods, health care referrals, and nutrition education for low-income pregnant, breastfeeding, and non-breastfeeding postpartum women, and to infants and children up to age five who are found to be at nutritional risk."[1] The clinic did a quick assessment and dispensed a can of powdered infant formula and instructed the mother on how to mix the formula. After a month or so, the baby's stooling pattern changed and the mother became concerned that the child was constipated. The mother returned with the baby to the WIC clinic. The staff evaluated the baby and told the mother that if she wanted liquid formula, her physician would have to order it for her. The mother then went to her physician. The mother informed us that the physician examined the child and said that everything was fine but he ordered the change in formula.

The child continued to have difficulty. The mother stated that the infant was not eating well, was fussy, and seemed to her to be uncomfortable. The mother asked a friend what to do. The friend suggested the mother give the child watered down manzanilla tea. Manzanilla is the Spanish term for chamomile. The mother tried the tea but the baby seemed to be increasingly uncomfortable. She bought over the counter infant gas drops for the child.

After trying the gas drops the mother became concerned that the child did not seem to be breathing right. She took the child to a local hospital emergency room. My understanding is that the child was seen by a nurse in the emergency room, and the nurse told the mother that there was nothing wrong with the child, that the mother was simply overreacting. Shortly thereafter the child had a respiratory and then cardiac arrest.

The child was immediately intubated: a breathing tube was inserted through her mouth into her windpipe. She was ventilated with a valve-equipped rubber bag and then placed on a ventilator. With the operating diagnosis of sepsis—that is, a blood infection—the child was then started on powerful antibiotics and transferred to the pediatric intensive care unit where she was currently hospitalized.

Over the intervening six days in the pediatric intensive care unit, the child failed to improve. The cultures taken of her blood, urine, and spinal fluid were all negative for bacteria and the staff was baffled as to what was going on when the child's breathing looked like she was gasping and her blood studies revealed a metabolic acidosis. That plus the history of the use of the infant gas medicine led to the call, and to saving the baby's life.

I learned a long time ago that although breast-fed babies can go through a phase that looks like constipation, they maintain their activity, eat well, and when they do have a stool it is loose. This baby fit the classical picture of a baby with infant botu-

---

[1] USDA United States Department of Agriculture Food and Nutrition Service, Women, Infants, and Children (WIC). http://www.fns.usda.gov/wic/women-infants-and-children-wic (accessed 29 March 2016).

lism, and I told the resident to get her attending immediately and arrange to purchase the antitoxin from California. We faxed the forms for the hospital to fill out with the history and told the resident to fax it to the California Department of Health's Infant Botulism division. We also faxed her the order form with the information on how to arrange payment and to expedite shipment. I told her that I would get to the hospital to see the child as soon as I could, but that I was hopelessly tied up with administrative and teaching responsibilities and not to hold off treatment.

The medicine is indeed costly; at that time the charge from the California Department of Health was $38,000.[2] It is impossible to put a price on an infant's life. But it is easy to say that without the treatment, if the child can be kept alive with the use of a ventilator, intravenous feedings, etc., the cost of the extended medical care required would exceed the price of the anti-toxin within five or ten days! The hospital was convinced quickly and the antitoxin ordered and administered. As expected the baby's response was rapid and amazing. Although the baby was still floppy, within hours she began breathing on her own, without the gasping movements that worried the resident so much. The following day, I was able to break away and our team of students and specialists travelled to see the child.

When we saw the child, she was definitely floppy. Her reflexes were difficult to ascertain. She had an incomplete startle response and no associated cry. Her mother was at the bedside and I was able to confirm the history that the resident gave me. In addition the mother told me that she had been experiencing pains in her nipples after about a week of nursing and she put an aloe cream on her breasts. That did not relieve the pain and then between that pain and the fact that the baby didn't seem to want to latch on, she was advised by her neighbor to smear honey onto her breasts, which she tried. She also told me about the chamomile tea. I asked her to bring in the bottle of honey and the tea so that I could get it analyzed. She said that she certainly would.

Unfortunately, the staff at the hospital had been unable to collect the needed stool specimen to test for botulinum. I was convinced of the diagnosis even without the laboratory confirmation, but I tried a digital rectal exam to stimulate a stool but this failed.

The child continued to improve. The mother did bring in the honey and tea. When I asked where they were, I was told that the nurses felt they were so dangerous, they threw them out!

The baby continued to make steady progress. At three weeks the child appeared alert, with good muscle tone, and, when offered a nipple from a bottle, gladly sucked it with great force. Three days after the anti-toxin was administered, the staff was finally able to collect a stool and sent it to the laboratory for analysis. At four weeks of admission, the New Jersey Department of Health informed us that they identified botulinum type A in the child's stools. The analysis is performed with sterilized stool injected into mice. The mice are pretreated with protective anti-toxin for a specific type of toxin, A, B and F, the most common forms of botulinum encountered

---

[2] Current purchase price is $45,300. State of California Health and Human Services. http://www. infantbotulism.org/physician/IPA-2013.pdf (accessed 29 March 2016).

in such cases. In this case the mice pretreated with anti-toxin A, lived while those pretreated with antitoxin to types B and F died.

Infant botulism, unlike botulism encountered in adults, is really an infectious process rather than simply an intoxication. To develop infant botulism the baby simply ingests spores of the bacteria. Botulinum spores are ubiquitous in nature and are very resistant to destruction by normal heat and other factors. An adult's normal stomach acid and other enzymes destroy these spores, as does high heat, under pressure, for example, in a pressure cooker or autoclave. A baby's stomach juices are not able to destroy the spores. In fact, the liquid environment and body temperature within the stomach enable the spores to germinate from spores to what are called vegetative forms. It is these vegetative forms which reproduce and produce the toxin which then causes the clinical effects. There is debate as to the importance of the use of antibiotics to terminate the growth of the vegetative forms. The use of certain antibiotics, called aminoglycosides, is often warned against, because they can cause paralysis of muscle function themselves.

Outbreaks of infant botulism occur each year. Interestingly there appears to be a distinct geographical distribution both in terms of number of cases and type of botulinum involved. Since the first cases were defined in California in 1976, over 80% of all cases were reported in the three states of California, Pennsylvania, and Utah. Additionally, most cases diagnosed on the East Coast are type B while most on the west coast are type A. One explanation for this geographical distribution is that botulinum type A survives better in neutral to alkaline soils while type B seems to do better in slightly acid soils.

The age distribution of infant botulism is remarkably similar to that of the Sudden Infant Death Syndrome (SIDS) and infant sepsis. When I checked with our state medical examiner, I discovered that they do not routinely screen for botulism in cases of SIDS. They feel that the presentation of SIDS is such that botulism would not be in the differential. I remarked on the apparent "risk factor" of breast feeding. I suggested that perhaps rather than being a risk factor, breast milk may protect the breast-fed baby from infant botulism and that breast-fed babies survive to be diagnosed while the bottle-fed baby die of SIDS. The medical examiner was not impressed.

The diagnosis of infant botulism is increasing worldwide. An article published in 2008 revealed the presence of significant contamination of chamomile products in Buenos Aires. The findings of such botulinum spores paralleled the findings in honey in the United States and led public health officials in Argentina to issue a warning to parents not to feed infants under one year of age any chamomile preparations, as the United States does for honey.

The botulinum toxin has been studied extensively. The "raw toxin" consists of two chains joined by a site that is subjected to cleavage. The heavy chains only function appears to be to help anchor the total toxin to the nerve cell membrane and allow the light chain to enter the cell. Once within the cell, the light chain appears to interfere with the docking mechanism, which enables tiny vesicles, or bags, containing the neurotransmitter acetylcholine, to move from the cytoplasm of the nerve cell and to anchor on the inner surface of the nerve cell. Once anchored the vesicle releases the acetylcholine into the space between the nerve ending and the muscle cell and causes the muscle to contract. Blocking this docking by the botulinum toxin results in the paralysis of that muscle's activity. If enough muscles are paralyzed, the individual cannot move and will eventually be unable to breathe. This mechanism is common to all forms of botulinum toxicity. The anti-toxin is capable of binding the toxin and preventing its effects. Theoretically then, once paralysis occurs, the anti-toxin will have little or no ability to reverse paralysis. That is the case with adults, and even after the antitoxin is administered it takes weeks, or even months, for motor function to return to normal. The observation in the infant in this case was the rapid regaining of muscle tone after the anti-toxin is administered is shared by many observers. It is unclear if there is a different docking mechanism in infants, if they can regrow the proteins needed to function in the docking action, or what other phenomenon is responsible for the dramatic improvement seen only in infants.

Preventive methods are the cornerstone of combating this disease. The United States American Academy of Pediatrics and the World Health Organization both warn against feeding any honey products to children before their first birthday. The Argentinian authorities extend this warning to chamomile products as well. Physicians warn their nursing mothers to wash their hands and their breasts with soap and water and to cook food appropriately.

One month after admission the baby was transferred to a children's rehabilitation hospital so that she could be monitored further and her swallowing improved through the intervention of therapists. She was discharged from that facility approximately a week later.

Suggested Reading

Arnon SS, Midura TF, Clay SA, et al. Infant botulism: epidemiological, clinical, and laboratory aspects. JAMA. 1977;237:1946–51.

Arnon SS, Schechter R, Maslanka SE, et al. Human botulinum immune globulin for the treatment of infant botulism. N Engl J Med. 2006;354:461–71.

Chapter 13
My Wife Is Trying to Kill Me!

It had already been a historic winter. The day after Christmas, heavy snows fell in the Northeast crippling the cities and towns of northern New Jersey and New York. It was now January 25 and northern New Jersey had just suffered through two weeks of arctic-like weather. On January 24 the temperature dropped to single digits. On the morning of January 25 the National Weather Service was predicting a day that would be mostly cloudy with a high of 36 degrees Fahrenheit and that light snow would start falling the following morning. The newscasters' prediction of the weather on every radio and television station was consistent as I relaxed at home the evening of the 25th. At some time that evening, as a precaution against another foul-up in the forecast, the New Jersey State Police issued a winter weather awareness alert for a potential winter storm the following day, January 26. The warning included the advisory that residents and commuters should prepare for the impending winter weather expected the following day and which could affect commuters. I had a New Jersey Drug Utilization Review Board (DURB) meeting scheduled for that morning. The DURB is a statewide committee established by the Department of Human Services to look into issues of medication utilization in various populations in the state covered by a state-sponsored medication program. I wondered whether I would be going to that meeting, obviously depending on what the weather would bring. I prepared to go to sleep early so that I could get up early in case the weather brought significant snowfall and I would need to make a decision on whether to attend the meeting or not. As my wife and I sat discussing what we would be doing the following day, a telephone call came from the New Jersey poison center. Diantha Clark, one of the nurse specialists in poison information, was on the line. She had received a call from an intensive care unit physician about a thirty-nine-year-old patient who had been in the hospital for eleven days. He was admitted for symptoms of gastritis, abdominal pain, vomiting, and diarrhea. He had eaten rice and beans for lunch, prepared by his wife, and developed the symptoms soon afterward. When seen in the emergency department he was complaining of severe abdominal pains and diarrhea. The physicians examining him made the tentative

© Springer International Publishing AG 2017
S.M. Marcus, *Medical Toxicology: Antidotes and Anecdotes*,
DOI 10.1007/978-3-319-51029-3_13

diagnosis of either an intestinal viral gastroenteritis or food poisoning with moderate dehydration. He was given intravenous fluids for the dehydration and admitted to the hospital.

Clark continued telling me what she had learned: over the next day his diarrhea improved but he developed strange neurological symptoms not usually seen with gastroenteritis. He complained of paresthesias—numbness, like pins and needles—which later evolved into excruciating pain in all of his extremities. The pain became so intense that he was refusing to move his legs, a pseudo-paralysis. The pain syndrome he developed is sometimes referred to as the "Little Mermaid Syndrome," the technical term in medicine is allodynia. In Hans Christian Andersen's story, when the little mermaid received her legs, she was left with nearly constant pain: "Every footstep felt as if she were walking on the blades and points of sharp knives."[1] Four days into the hospitalization, he developed some weakness of his lower extremities. A neurological consultation was obtained and it was felt that he might have Guillain-Barré Syndrome. This syndrome consists of a peculiar constellation of neurological symptoms and signs including an ascending paralysis of muscles. It does not usually include the strange sensory defects that this patient demonstrated. Guillain-Barré often occurs after a viral infection, but its etiology is truly unknown. (A variety of the syndrome mimics the potentially deadly poisoning with the toxin botulism, but that was not considered in this case, since in botulism the initial paralysis is usually in muscles involved with swallowing and progresses downward rather than upward.) The physicians, however, believed that the diagnosis of Guillain-Barré was "confirmed" by the finding of an elevation of protein in his spinal fluid, and he was treated for five days with immune gamma globulin, a preparation made from human blood which contains antibodies which has been shown to be efficacious in such cases.

The continued existence of sensory findings led the neurological consultant to suggest that a "urine screen" for "heavy metal" poisonings be obtained. The screen generally includes testing for lead, arsenic, and mercury as the most commonly encountered heavy metals. Four days after submitting the urine, the results were reported as negative. At about that same time, the patient started having seizures. When the seizures occurred, he was transferred to the intensive care unit. When the nurses discussed the case, one nurse stated that she had recently read of a poisoning case in China which was caused by the metal thallium and she thought that their patient's symptoms were like those in the Chinese case. She stated that since the patient at their hospital was Chinese, perhaps it could be the same metal. The physicians then called the laboratory, which luckily still had the urine sample, and agreed to "add on" the test for thallium. Prompting the call to the poison center was the report from the laboratory of an extremely high level of thallium. Diantha asked if I would speak to the attending physician at the hospital.

---

[1] Hans Christian Andersen, "The Little Mermaid" ("Den lille Havfrue"), translated by Jean Hersholt, *The Complete Andersen* (New York: Limited Editions Club, 1949). Available on the website of the Hans Christian Andersen Center at the University of Southern Denmark, http://www.andersen.sdu.dk/vaerk/hersholt/TheLittleMermaid:e.html (accessed 5 May 2016).

Dr. Thon Pai (a pseudonym) and I began to discuss the case. As soon as he confirmed the finding of thallium in the urine, my initial comment was that the hospital should alert law-enforcement because the only cases of thallium poisoning that I knew of were either suicides or murders. At that point Dr. Pai asked if I had been consulted before and I said no. Dr. Pai stated that the patient, on admission, stated that he thought his wife was trying to kill him. Dr. Pai stated that the staff felt the patient was simply paranoid. In fact a psychiatric consultation had been obtained and recorded the belief that the patient was expressing paranoid ideation but the psychiatrist "guessed the possibility should be explored." My comment after hearing that was that they definitely needed to contact the County Prosecutor's office, since it is that law enforcement team which gets involved in capital or potentially capital crimes. We discussed the nature of the gentleman's paresthesias and that the patient complained of needle sharp pains with such a severity that he was not moving around in his bed. The physician reported that there had been no hair loss, a cardinal sign of thallium poisoning usually presenting about two weeks after the poisoning.

I suggested to Dr. Pai that the institution look for the antidote, Prussian blue. I stated that there might be some in the hospital pharmacy as part of the stockpile for use in bioterrorism, particularly radiation exposures. I also stated that they might have some non-medicinal Prussian blue in the pathology laboratory, since it is used as a histology dye. I also suggested that the hospital reach out to the New Jersey Department of Health and Senior Services to see if the state might expedite receipt of Prussian blue from the national stockpile for bioterrorism. I knew that Prussian blue was available at Oak Ridge National Laboratory and suggested that the hospital reach out to their Radiation Emergency Assistance Center/Training Site (REACTS). I advised that they start, immediately, by administering activated charcoal. Thallium can be "recycled" from the blood through the liver's biliary tree, the gall bladder and biliary ducts, into the intestine where it can be absorbed again into the bloodstream. This is called entero-hepatic recycling. Charcoal is administered in an attempt to bind any thallium that might be in the intestine or could be pulled from the blood through the gastrointestinal tract, or could be recycled through the liver into the intestine until Prussian blue became available. Prussian blue's therapeutic efficacy is thought to be similar: the binding of thallium in the intestinal lumen.

The following morning I awakened a little earlier than usual, at 5:00 a.m., to prepare for my morning exercises and commute. When I peeked out the window I saw that a significant amount of snow had already fallen and that the snowplows had plowed the street in front of my house but had not cleared my driveway. I lived in a condominium community which takes care of plowing the roads and cleaning the snow from driveways and sidewalks. The priority is to clear the roads and then get to the driveways when manpower is available. I knew that they would eventually get to my driveway, but had no idea when that would happen. Considering that I would have to go either to the DURB meeting and or the hospital (the hospital was located a short distance from the location of the DURB meeting), I decided to skip my normal morning workout routine and got dressed to do snow removal. I spent the next hour or so getting the snow off of my driveway so that I could get my car, which luckily was an all-wheel drive vehicle, out of my driveway and onto the street. I believed that if I could get out of my development, I would have a good chance of reaching the location of the DURB or the hospital. Listening to the news, it sounded as if it was going to be a white-knuckle trip most of the way in. A call from the hospital pharmacy buyer at 7:45 a.m. revealed that she had been unable to locate any prussian blue. I was just about to leave and attempt the voyage and suggested that she reach out to the Department of Health and consider calling REACTS. At the same time, I reached out to Christopher Rinn, the Assistant Commissioner of the New Jersey Department of Health and Senior Services (NJDHSS) for emergency preparedness and explained the story to him. I told him that I believed that Prussian blue, used in treating victims of "dirty bombs," is in the federal stockpile of materials to use in bioterrorism events. I didn't know how we could arrange to access it and asked him to attempt to gain access to the antidote. Mr. Rinn assured me that I had the full cooperation of the NJDHSS with respect to locating and delivering the medication to the patient's bedside.

A call to the hospital determined that the patient was now in extremely poor condition. He was in shock and was now on a mechanical ventilator. My car's Bluetooth connectivity enabled me to field calls as I drove. I received a telephone call from Dr. Christiansen of Oak Ridge National Laboratories informing me that Oak Ridge had received clearance from the Department of Energy to ship the drug and, barring any difficulty because of the snowstorm, it was felt that the drug should reach the hospital sometime that evening. He stated that they would ship ninety capsules of 500 mg each. The resident at the hospital called the poison center to report that the patient's blood pressure had dropped to dangerous levels and he needed medication to support his blood pressure, and also that his kidneys were showing signs of failing. Shortly thereafter, the hospital's clinical pharmacist called and reported that she found some technical grade (not meant for human consumption) Prussian blue and agreed to start using it. We discussed how to dose it, and, since it was not medicinal grade, we simply took the usual suggested dose and decided to administer twice that amount. I suggested that nephrology be on board and consider dialysis in an effort to sustain him.

I received a call from Joe Kolakowski of the NJDHSS. He worked in Mr. Rinn's program and was confirming that he had located some Prussian blue in a storage depot in New York State. He arranged for it to be transported in a relay, first by New York State Police, then transferred, at the New Jersey border, to the New Jersey State Police and would be delivered sometime that morning or early afternoon to the hospital. It was snowing too badly for a helicopter to transport it, and they had no idea how long it would take to reach the hospital from the depot in the snowstorm.

Arriving at the hospital I was greeted by a member of the hospital's security team in the parking lot. Somehow he recognized that this crazy lunatic out in the blizzard must be Dr. Marcus. He escorted me into the hospital and I was greeted by detectives from the two different county prosecutors' offices (the victim lived in a different county from the hospital and representatives of both counties' prosecutor's offices were present) who were anxious to hear information about thallium. We had a lengthy discussion about the poison before I was able to leave them and proceed to the bedside to help treat the patient.

The hospital was a beautiful example of brick-faced hospital architecture, which looked at home in the revolutionary-era style architecture of its surrounding community. The intensive care unit was designed in classic nineties design with rooms too small to house all of the modern equipment needed to treat critically ill patients. When I walked into the unit, I had to sidestep equipment stored in the spaces between patient areas, to gain access to the alcove-like space in which the patient was being cared for. There was so much equipment surrounding him that I had a great deal of difficulty getting to him. He was attached to multiple intravenous infusion lines, and had a large breathing tube in his mouth connected by tubing to a bedside mechanical ventilator. A tube was taped to his nose and drained fluid into a suction apparatus hanging on the wall. He was attached by tubing to a dialysis machine. Wires attached to his chest were connected to monitoring equipment which displayed his heart and respiratory rate. Tubing in an artery in his arm was attached to a device which would then send information to his monitor and display his blood pressure. Each of the machines had their own distinct sound; the result was a virtual symphony, from the steady beat of the ventilator to the beeping of his heart rate. Around the bed was an army of nurses, physicians, and students either directly involved in his care or anxious to learn about thallium poisoning.

The residents and attending met with me to review the case. We walked away from the bedside so that we could discuss the case in more comfortable quarters. The lead resident presented the case to me. "This thirty-nine-year-old Asian male with no significant past medical history presented to the emergency department stating that he thought someone was poisoning him. He had acute onset abdominal pain, which began one to two hours after eating lunch consisting of homemade rice and green beans. The pain was described as dull, progressing in intensity. He also complained of multiple bouts of diarrhea. He denied any presence of blood in his stool. He denied any vomiting but stated that he was nauseated. He apparently drove himself to the hospital."[2] The resident continued with his presentation, "According to his wife, their child was recently hospitalized with a similar illness. His wife ingested the same food, had some diarrhea but no pain."

The resident continued his presentation: "Family history was positive for dyslipidemia [abnormalities in the fat content of his blood, such as cholesterol]. His past medical history was negative. Social history obtained, four days after admission, revealed that the husband and wife had filed for divorce in July 2010 and the final court date was the day of his admission. The patient stated that his wife was a chemist and that he suspected that she may be poisoning him."

"Physical examination on admission to the ED revealed vital signs: pulse 63 bpm, BP 137/89, RR 20. General physical exam was negative including his abdominal examination. Initial laboratory evaluation showed normal blood count, electrolytes, and liver functions. Abdominal ultrasound was normal as was a CAT scan of his abdomen and pelvis.

---

[2] The dialogues here were recreated from notes I took at the time and placed onto the electronic medical record of the poison center.

"Later, on the day of admission, he began complaining of hypoesthesias (partial loss of sensation; diminished sensibility), describing the feeling of pins and needles in his extremities. The report of the neurological consultation revealed a slightly different history in that the patient stated to the neurologist that two days prior to the admission he started having bilateral parasthesias (a skin sensation, such as burning, prickling, itching, or tingling, with no apparent physical cause) of his hands and then a day later developed *painful* paresthesias of his feet. These parasthesias progressed during the hospital stay as did his abdominal pain. He further developed fluctuating levels of alertness. Eventually the paresthesias became so bad that he could not or would not move his legs. The neurologist considered the diagnosis of Guillain-Barré Syndrome and he received intravenous immune globulin (a blood product which contains antibodies for various illnesses and is often found helpful in this condition) with no relief of symptomatology."

The team then shared with me the fact that, according to the history obtained by a consulting psychiatrist, during the fifth hospital day, the patient claimed he had an episode of paresthesias around Thanksgiving of 2010. According to what the treatment team told me then, the psychiatrist questioned him about his comment that he thought his wife was poisoning him, to which he responded that the fact that he became so sick the day the divorce was finalized was just too much of a coincidence. The resident then told us that the psychiatrist commented in his note, "He [the patient] apparently has been requesting to have his urine tested for possible poisoning." The psychiatrist stated in his summary that it was "difficult to see whether he qualifies for a psychiatric diagnosis. Nonetheless, the fact that he is accusing his wife of poisoning him may suggest the presence of a paranoid syndrome, although one has to first exclude the possibility of any kind of poisoning, and urine studies are pending."[3]

The resident continued, "On the third hospital day, the neurologist suggested obtaining a twenty-four-hour urine for heavy metal screen.[4] The result of the lead, mercury, and arsenic came back as negative on the tenth hospital day. On the eighth hospital day, he was found actively seizing and required large doses of anticonvulsive medication. He required intubation to protect his airway and to provide ventilation. It was at this point that he was transferred to the ICU and a nurse told the doctors that she had read of a case of thallium poisoning in China and she suggested that since the victim and his wife were both Chinese, perhaps thallium might have been used in the poisoning of the victim. The hospital called the laboratory in Minnesota and added thallium to the tests."

The attending physician, present for the discussion, then explained that on the day of the call to the poison center, on the twelfth hospital day, the result of his twenty-four hour urine collection became available. The victim had voided 4300 mL

---

[3] The resident read the information directly from the chart and I was able to review the chart and confirm these statements.

[4] I have never been able to find a good definition of heavy metal, but generally the term is used to describe such metals as lead, mercury, and arsenic while light metals refer to lithium and titanium.

of urine (most adults don't produce that amount unless their kidneys are unable to concentrate the urine or they receive or drink much too much fluid) during the twenty-four hour period and although the analysis was negative for lead and arsenic, the thallium level was reported as >800 mcg/L, a truly remarkable finding, since there should never be any thallium in the urine. At around the same time he developed hypotension, shock, and that was when the poison center was consulted.

The attending stated that the poison center suggested starting multiple dose activated charcoal, keeping his serum potassium high, repeating the urine testing and obtaining a blood for thallium level confirmation. She reminded us that since he was so symptomatic the poison center suggested empirical therapy with Prussian blue, the suggested antidote. The resident then chimed in, "The poison center, and our pharmacy helped us find some Prussian blue. The following morning, he needed pressor support to keep his mean arterial blood pressure over 50."

At the end of the presentation, a young woman in scrubs and a white coat approached me. She introduced herself as the clinical pharmacist and said she was there to work with me in anyway needed. She had helped administer the technical grade antidote and was anticipating receipt of the supply of medicinal grade preparation from Albany.

I did a cursory examination of the patient. It was difficult to get around his bed to examine him, the space was so occupied with medical equipment. He lacked some of the expected physical findings of thallium poisoning. One of the hallmarks of the poisoning is the loss of hair. He had relatively thin scalp hair, but it did not come out of his scalp upon gentle pulling. Hair loss characteristically occurs approximately two weeks after an exposure to thallium. I examined his nail beds and there were no Mees' lines. Mees' lines also known as Aldrich–Mees' lines, or *leukonychia* striata, are horizontal lines of discoloration across the nails of the fingers and toes. Mees' lines are more often associated with chronic exposures and appear over time. The only external abnormality I did notice was a change in his skin texture, specifically that of his scrotum. The skin was thick and parchment-like, suggesting a degree of hyperkeratosis, or thickening of the surface layer of the skin, a very peculiar finding in that region where skin is usually so thin and pliable.

The staff gathered around me as if expecting to hear extraordinary words of wisdom. I started by explaining that thallium was once used as a rat poisoning, but its severe toxicity when ingested by children and pets led to its removal from licensing for use in the United States. My own experiences with a person poisoned with thallium consisted of two cases that I consulted on directly. In one case, a school teacher developed total loss of hair and had an elevated level of thallium in her urine. There were several teachers in her school with a variety of strange symptoms and signs all consistent with thallium exposure, but none suffered from more than hair loss. Neither public health officials nor law enforcement was ever able to establish a cause of their exposure. The problem disappeared as mysteriously as it had appeared. The other case involved a man exposed to thallium through his job making a salt of thallium for a chemical supply company. I was peripherally involved with a third case proven to be related to thallium poisoning; a professor at New York University attempted to poison a federal judge who had sentenced him to jail for using his university laboratory to manufacture illicit drugs. The professor sent a box of chocolates, which were laced with thallium, to the judge's home. The judge's wife ate a few candies and collapsed.[5] I also knew of a case in Florida in which an entire family suffered when a neighbor added thallium to cola soda they stored on their back porch. That episode was memorialized in the book *Poison Mind*, by Jeffrey Good and Susan Goreck. There was a famous outbreak of poisoning from malicious use of the poison. In the 1940s and 1950s an outbreak of thallium poisonings occurred in Australia, the result of the use of the poison by some women who murdered their husbands, neighbors, and others.[6]

Thallium, which masquerades as the essential mineral potassium, enters the body from the gastrointestinal tract and, in some forms, even through the skin. The metal enters into tissues through essential mineral channels and poisons the body by taking the place of potassium in vital organ tissues and chemical reactions. The only treatment, I explained, was the use of hemodialysis to remove whatever thallium is circulating in the blood, and administering Prussian blue to bind thallium in the intestine and enhance the gastrointestinal elimination. Once patients become symptomatic, it is unlikely that even the antidote will be successful.

Shortly after the discussion, another pharmacist came into the ICU with a bottle of Radiogardase®, ferric ferrocyanide, medicinal-grade Prussian blue. This medicine—approved for treating exposure to radioactive cesium, the potential radioactive component of a dirty bomb—is the only reported antidote for thallium poisoning. The pills had made the trip from the storage depot in New York, through the driving snow, in less than three hours, a trip which usually takes about four hours in good weather.

The clinical pharmacist and I went to the pharmacy to mix up the solution we would administer via the tube in the patient's stomach. We were startled by the beauty of the capsules. Neither of us had ever seen the pure medicinal dye before and were in awe of what we had before us. Carefully mixing it into solution we then returned to the bedside.

Shortly after the drug was administered, the patient's vital signs deteriorated. We then administered increased intravenous fluids and medications to strengthen his heart beat and blood pressure. We were losing ground. A new mode of therapy for overdoses involving medications which decrease heart beat strength was being suggested for a variety of agents. After a brief discussion, we administered an infusion of a 20% suspension of lipid emulsion. The theory was that the preparation would be absorbed by heart tissue and provide added energy to enhance the contraction of his heart. Unfortunately, we did not see any change in the trend in his vital signs,

---

[5] Lubasch A. "Professor Pleades Guilty in Poisoned Candy Case," *New York Times*, 10 June 1987. http://www.nytimes.com/1987/06/10/nyregion/professor-pleads-guilty-in-poisoned-candy-case.html (accessed 7 May 2016).

[6] The Australian TV documentary *Recipe for Murder* (dir. Sonia Bible), released in 2011, examines three of the most sensational and widely-reported Australian thallium poisonings: the Fletcher, Monty, and Grills cases. For a review of the film, see Tim Elliott, "Recipe For Murder: The Poisoners' Tales," *Sydney Morning Herald*, 22 May 2011, http://www.smh.com.au/entertainment/tv-and-radio/recipe-for-murder-the-poisoners-tales-20110520-1evcj.html (accessed 5 May 2016).

heart rate or blood pressure. As we all gathered around him in attempting to resuscitate him, all we saw was his cardiac rhythm "straight line." After all of the intensive efforts, we were too late in our intervention and his life slipped away.

There was a woman sitting at the patient's bedside. I asked who she was, and was told she was his wife, and that she had been at his bedside off and on since admission. I was informed that she had even fed him food from home while he was in the hospital. This was the very person that the patient said he thought was trying to kill him. This fact kept haunting me all of the way back to my office from the hospital. When I arrived at my office, I went directly to the computer to see whether it was possible to order any thallium online. I was amazed at how easily I was able to find a supplier, one that was in fact located in New Jersey, and I went right up to the point of ordering the substance before I stopped.

The next day, a case worker from the New Jersey children's protective services, the Division of Youth and Family Service (DYFS), called my office requesting information. He believed that that the son of the couple had been admitted to another hospital two weeks prior to the presentation of the victim. He was asking if there was any way to prove that there might have been any abuse related to that admission. I explained that it would be unlikely that there was any specimen left from that date but that I would call and find out if the hospitalization caused any "red flags." I called an old friend of mine at the hospital the case worker mentioned, its director of pediatrics, and requested he look to see if there was any record of a child with that last name, particularly looking to see if there might have been anything suspicious that went unreported. He later called back to say that he couldn't find anything. I reached out to a medical toxicologist at another hospital in the same city as the one reported by the DYFS worker, and she found no child by that name.

Two days after the death, I received a telephone call from an investigator with the county prosecutor's office. He related to me that the victim and his wife had a history of domestic abuse. In March 2010, nine months prior to the current events, the victim claimed he was being poisoned by his wife and gave the police a sample of milk that he believed she had poisoned. This milk was never tested, and was still with the police. The couple filed for divorce in July. The investigator stated that wife worked in arthritis research at a large pharmaceutical manufacturer. It was determined by the investigator that she ordered thallium chloride outside of the usual ordering system at her company and requisitioned it. Sometime after she ordered and requisitioned the thallium, she reported to her local police department that she believed her husband was trying to poison her with something in her tea. She gave them a sample, although it had not yet been analyzed. She repeatedly called to see if they had the results. She returned the thallium chloride to the storeroom at her company on Dec 10, 2010. The seal had been changed and very little of the substance had been "unaccounted for," but the substance in the container had not been analyzed. The final divorce decree was issued on January 10, 2011, the day the patient presented at the hospital with diarrhea. According to the prosecutor's office, the nurses reported that, while in the hospital, the wife brought in "soup" from home which she fed the victim while he was in the hospital. Hazmat executed a search warrant and removed various powders and other materials from the couple's home.

On that same day another investigator, told me that DYFS informed the mother that she had to take her two-year-old son for testing; otherwise, he would be removed from her custody pending outcome of the investigation. A detective from the New Jersey State Police called to ask if I knew of anyone who would be able to examine the various food items for thallium. I suggested National Medical Services and Atlantic Diagnostic Laboratories but found an article discussing a Florida case in which the Federal Bureau of Investigation's laboratory apparently analyzed Coca-Cola for thallium and this was what was used in court (this was the same case that I mentioned as described in the book *The Poison Mind*). I gave the detective the name of a clinical toxicologist, a doctoral-trained pharmacist I knew from attending national meetings, with special training and certification in applied toxicology who was working in a laboratory at the FBI in Quantico, Virginia. The investigator asked if I had any explanation for why the specific preparation thallium chloride might have been used. I could only guess that since that is the salt used in thallium stress tests, a common test of heart function, if the substance was found in his body, his wife might have tried to claim that he had a recent stress test. That ploy would probably not have worked because the stress test dose is far less than what would have been the dose used to kill him. I reached out to an old toxicology friend, a pharmacist who ran a poison center in Michigan and had an international reputation as a forensic toxicologist, to see if he could come up with something better and he said my guess was possibly the best.

As reported in the *Star-Ledger*, the major newspaper of the state of New Jersey: "forty year old chemist Tianle Li stood before a judge in New Brunswick on Wednesday and listened with quiet composure as she was charged with murdering her husband by dosing him with a rare lethal substance. Li's lawyer, Steven Altman, entered a plea of not guilty, and a few minutes later, the hearing was over."[7]

In that same article, the *Star-Ledger* included information about our attempt to obtain the Prussian blue. Included in the report was the fact that I had dug myself out from the snow to get my car out of my garage so that I could drive to the hospital. I was castigated by the community's management firm for embarrassing the community and was told that anytime I need to get out, in a valid emergency, I should call and they would clear my driveway as a priority.

The trial, which commenced more than two years after the fatal events occurred, lasted almost two months and as reported again in the Star Ledger: "Just as she had throughout her murder trial, Tianle Li sat stoically as the guilty verdict was read." "The jury convicted the forty four year old former chemist at Bristol-Myers Squibb of fatally poisoning her husband in January 2011 with thallium, a tasteless, odorless and highly lethal drug, after he had sought a divorce."[8]

---

[7] "Doctors, scientists searched for antidote for Monroe man dying from thallium poisoning," Star ledger. **Posted on line** on February 10, 2011 at 7:15 a.m., updated February 10, 2011 at 8:40 a.m. http://www.nj.com/news/index.ssf/2011/02/doctors_scientists_led_heroic.html   accessed   29 Marcy 2016.

[8] Epstein Sue. "Jury Convicts Monroe Woman of Poisoning Her Husband." NJ Advance Media (formerly The Star Ledger) posted on July 09, 2013 at 2:20 p.m., updated July 10, 2013 at 6:26 a.m.

The newspaper later reported that Li, a Chinese citizen, was sentenced to life in prison without release until 85% of the term is served, or at least sixty-two years, six months and nineteen days in prison.[9]

More than three years after the death, I was finally able to obtain a copy of the post mortem examination. There was nothing to see on the gross or microscopic evaluation except for some "congestion" of the victim's organs. The toxicology done on various body tissues was startling. Blood concentrations of thallium ranged from a low of 1400 mcg/L to a high of 5000 mcg/L. There was thallium found in the gastric fluid at 220 mcg/L and thallium was found in his hair from 1.6 to 4.6 mcg/g. Urine retained from the hospital revealed thallium concentration of 19,000 mcg/L, but when corrected for creatinine in the urine, a way to estimate a 24 h elimination of thallium, the result popped the top of the credibility level at 57,000 mcg of thallium per gram of creatinine. Those levels will probably be the highest I will ever see.

Suggested Reading

Cvjetko P, Cvjetko I, Pavlica M. Thallium toxicity in humans. Arh Hig Rada Toksikol. 2010;61:111–9.

Good J, Goreck S. Poison mind: the true story of the mensa murderer-and the policewoman who risked her life to bring him to justice. William Morrow & Company: New York City; 1995.

Miller MA, Patel MM, Coon T. Prussian blue for treatment of thallium overdose in the US. Hosp Pharm. 2005;40(9).796–7.

Tsai YT, Huang CC, Kuo HC, et al. Central nervous system effects in acute thallium poisoning. Neurotoxicology. 2006;27:291–5.

Zhao G, Ding M, Zhang B, et al. Clinical manifestations and management of acute thallium poisoning. Eur Neurol. 2008;60:292–7.

Accessed 29 March 2016. http://www.nj.com/middlesex/index.ssf/2013/07/jury_resumes_deliberations_in_murder_trial_of_monroe_woman_charged_with_poisoning_her_husband.html

[9] Epstein, Sue. "N.J. woman sentenced to life in prison for fatally poisoning husband with thallium." NJ Advance Media (formerly The Star Ledger) posted on 30 September 2013: http://www.nj.com/middlesex/index.ssf/2013/09/nj_woman_sentenced_to_life_in_prison_for_fatally_poisoning_husband_with_thallium.html

Chapter 14
Torch Song

Pregnancy is an exciting time for a couple. They dream about their future family, imagine a happy chubby baby. Far from their minds is that something could alter the future of the baby. They repress such thoughts if they occur. This is true of all pregnancies, but by the time a couple is on their third child, thoughts for preparedness are not as detailed. So if the unfortunate happens, it can be devastating.

Baby boy V was born at thirty-seven weeks gestation to a thirty-one-year-old mother, the result of her third pregnancy. The pregnancy was uneventful and there was no expectation of any problem. The mother had the usual prenatal care. The baby was born via a normal spontaneous vaginal delivery weighing about 3 kg (about six-and-a-half pounds) at birth. Shortly after birth, the baby was noted to have petechiae, blood spots, all over his body. He was described as looking somewhat like a "blueberry muffin." He was sent to the neonatal intensive care unit for treatment. His stay in the intensive care unit was complicated by a decrease in platelets, the formed elements in the blood that aid in clot formation and prevention of bleeding. Such a decrease can present with the rash that he was demonstrating. He required multiple transfusions of platelets during his stay to restore his platelet function.

The presentation with a blueberry-like rash was suggestive of a child with the TORCH Syndrome. This is a mnemonic used to describe a group of congenital infections which present with similar findings. Those diseases are **TO**xoplasmosis, **R**ubella, **C**ytomegalovirus, and **H**erpes. Routine laboratory testing performed prior to his birth were negative for cytomegalovirus, herpes, syphilis, and hepatitis. He was found to have positive IgM and IgG serology for toxoplasmosis. Further testing of the mother after the neonate was found to be positive also revealed positive toxoplasmosis IgM and IgG serology. These facts supported the diagnosis of gestationally acquired toxoplasmosis with the resultant congenital infection of the infant. Opthalmological evaluation performed in the neonatal intensive care unit revealed

© Springer International Publishing AG 2017
S.M. Marcus, *Medical Toxicology: Antidotes and Anecdotes*,
DOI 10.1007/978-3-319-51029-3_14

that the patient had chorioretinitis, an inflammation of a part of the retina of the eye. There are various viruses which have been associated with chorioretinitis, but toxoplasmosis is by far the most common cause. It is believed that the majority of cases of acute toxoplasmic chorioretinitis in adults is the late sequelae of congenital infection, making the treatment in the neonatal period extremely important. Untreated this can lead to blindness. An MRI of the brain was negative for any structural abnormalities. Often infants with congenital toxoplasmosis have intracranial calcium deposition. The triad of chorioretinitis, hydrocephalus, and intracranial calcification is classically considered diagnostic. Using that as the diagnostic tool would miss cases, such as baby V, who did not present with the full triad. Baby V was "lucky" in that the diagnosis was made early and treatment begun immediately. This may have prevented the development of the other part of the triad. The diagnosis of congenital toxoplasmosis should be considered in infants who present with fever, intrauterine growth retardation, chorioretinitis, vomiting, bleeding (from puncture sites or petechaie, as in baby V), jaundice, hepatomegaly, splenomegaly, seizures, or other findings suggestive of neonatal infection.

The infant was started on pyrimethamine and sulfadiazine daily, and leucovorin three times a week.

Toxoplasmosis is said, by the United States Centers for Disease Control and Prevention (CDC), to be the second most common foodborne infectious disease resulting in fatalities, the first being salmonella. It is a not an uncommon infection, said to infect over one billion people worldwide. In studies of sero-prevalence in the United Kingdom, 7% of individuals are found to be positive for the antibody and therefore felt to have been infected. In the Central African Republic it is said that 80% of the population is seropositive, while the National Health and Nutrition Examination Study (NHANES) found a seroprevalence of toxoplasmosis in the United States of over 15 in the 13–49 age group. Seroprevalence in Europe is 54% in seven Southern European countries and decreases to 5%–10% in northern Sweden and Norway.

The CDC labels toxoplasmosis as a "neglected" infection. Such infections are considered as neglected because relatively little attention is devoted to its surveillance, prevention, and treatment.

Toxoplasmosis is an obligate intracellular parasite, unable to exist outside of an infected cell. It has three infectious stages: (1) the tachyzoite, the form responsible for the rapid spread of the parasite between cells and tissues and the clinical manifestations of toxoplasmosis; (2) bradyzoites, cysts contained within tissue, which maintain a chronic infection staying dormant for the life of the host unless the host becomes immunocompromised, at which point the cyst may mature and become infectious; (3) sporozoites contained within oocysts that are shed by members of the felid (cat) family in their stools. Cats are natural intermediaries in the lifecycle of toxoplasmosis. Individuals that have kittens in the house have greater incidences of infection with toxoplasmosis. The use of a litter box by a pet cat can become a hazard when people clean the litter and fail to wash properly before eating, or before putting their fingers into their mouth. These oocysts have been reported to be found in untreated water, in soil, on fruit and in raw shellfish.

The disease is transmitted in several different ways; horizontally through ingestion of contaminated water or soil, or the ingestion of meat containing the sporozoites. Vertical transmission is when an infected mother, infected somewhat late in her pregnancy, transmits the parasite through the placenta to the child. There have also been reports of transmission of toxoplasmosis through organ donation and blood transfusions. Additionally, there are reports of individual cases associated with eating raw ground beef, rare lamb, and locally produced, cured dry smoked meat; drinking unpasteurized goat milk; or eating raw oysters clams or mussels.

Congenital toxoplasmosis was first officially reported in 1938 when the organism was definitively identified in an infant girl delivered full-term by cesarean section and who developed convulsions and lesions in both eyes. The patient died in infancy and on postmortem examination, the organism was identified. This confirmed that the parasite was capable of crossing the placenta and that there was vertical transmission. The transplacental rate of transmission from an infected woman is between 60% and 90%. The severity of illness depends on the stage of gestation at the time of the infection and the extent of infection of the mother. It is said that congenital toxoplasmosis occurs in one in 10,000 live births. In the United States, it is believed that the clinical illness is seen in 400 cases annually. In France the incidence rate is 2.9 cases per 10,000 live births roughly three times that of the United States. The majority of these cases are asymptomatic or only mildly symptomatic. Congenital toxoplasmosis can result in fetal death if the infection is severe. It can produce a multitude of congenital abnormalities such as hydrocephalus (water on the brain), brain or hepatic calcifications, enlargement of the spleen, inflammation of the tissue surrounding the heart, intrauterine growth retardation, and hepatic injury producing fluid in the abdominal cavity. As in baby V, newborns can present with the typical rash described as blueberry muffin baby syndrome from the bleeding in the skin, petechial lesions. Babies may be small for gestational age, some may have microcephaly, small heads, while others may actually have large heads if the infection is severe enough to produce hydrocephalus. Babies may develop seizures, may have pneumonia, and may manifest other signs of infection such as jaundice and decreased platelet count. Blindness may result from the characteristic chorioretinitis and in addition there may be hearing loss.

The diagnosis is often made in the newborn period, generally on the basis of the constellation of symptoms with confirmatory serology. The difficulty with serological proof is that the mother might have been infected before gestation and carry a positive serology that will be transmitted to the baby and would not necessarily represent newborn infection. The most significant serology is a test for acute infection, elevations in immunoglobulin A (IgA). In general, babies usually present as if they have sepsis, unknown infection, and testing for TORCH is sent out to the laboratory as well as standard bacteriological testing for various bacteria and viruses in the affected baby. Depending on the results of preliminary testing, the child may be started on antibiotics for unknown sepsis. If the testing for TORCH returns positive, the antibiotic coverage would be changed to cover the treatment of this parasite.

There appears to be no way to distinguish infections caused by transmission from cats from the infections caused by ingesting infected meat or other sources. In a study done in Norway, eating raw or undercooked meat and meat products, poor kitchen hygiene, cleaning the cat litter box, and eating unwashed harvest vegetables or fruits were associated with increased risk of toxoplasmosis. A study in Italy revealed that in infected women who became infected during pregnancy, the greatest risk was eating cured pork or raw meat at least once a month. In a another European study the contact with raw or undercooked beef, lamb, or other meat as well as soil were independent risk factors for seroconversion during pregnancy

The majority of infections are subclinical and there is debate on the utility of screening pregnant women for infections. In some locations prenatal screening programs are in place and the conversion from zero negativity to IgM and IgG positive sera positivity forms a basis for the diagnosis. Low levels of toxoplasma-specific IgM antibodies can be found for up to several years after an acute infection in the presentation of low concentrations of Toxoplasma. The presence of IgM antibodies is therefore not regarded as an indication of an acute infection. It is sometimes difficult to make the diagnosis of an infection in a pregnant women when routine surveillance is not maintained on pregnant women.

Molecular testing with polymerize chain reaction, PCR, is considered the "gold standard" for the diagnosis of in-utero infection. With this technique, sensitivity may be as high as 100% but this is dependent on the gestational age at the time of the infection and when the blood is drawn. Sensitivity is also dependent upon the specific genetic subtype of toxoplasmosis.

IgM and IgA antibodies do not appear to cross the placenta and therefore the presence in the newborn suggests congenital infection. Neonatal screening programs are based on the detection of IgM antibodies in blood spots drawn routinely in all newborns for testing for inborn errors of metabolism, such as phenylketonuria, PKU. In some studies treatment of acute maternal toxoplasmosis during pregnancy eliminates or reduces the duration of the specific IgM response of the infant and is felt to demonstrate the protective effect of therapy.

Austria introduced the mandatory free monthly serological screening of pregnant women for toxoplasmosis in 1975. In the United States, Massachusetts and New Hampshire have mandatory newborn screening for toxoplasmosis.[1] Parts of Brazil, Denmark, and Ireland also have mandatory newborn screening for toxoplasmosis. In countries and places where mandatory screening is performed it is generally customary to start therapy as early as possible using different antibiotics depending on the stage of the infection in an attempt to decrease the potential damage from the infection to the developing fetus.

Treatment of children with congenitally acquired toxoplasmosis with pyrimethamine and sulfadiazine is the standard of care. It appears from long-term studies that the treatment of children symptomatic from congenital toxoplasmosis has improved outcome while in administering such therapy in asymptomatic children the improvement in outcome is not clear.

---

[1] For more about newborn screening, see http://www.babysfirsttest.org/newborn-screening/about-newborn-screening (accessed 30 March 2016).

Preventive efforts are suggested by most public health professionals. Since cats are a primary host, the existence in the house or stray cats in the environment is to be avoided. A job or activity that puts a pregnant woman in contact with soil, sand or other material which may have been contaminated by cat feces also puts her at risk.

The goal of treatment is to arrest the replication of the parasite and stop the progression of the disease and, if possible, to prevent permanent damage to the involved organs. The treatment for toxoplasmosis is based upon the fact that the parasite requires the production of proteins in order to reproduce and continue to survive. The production of such protein requires the activation of the vitamin folic acid to its active form, reduced folate, aka folinic acid. Treatment consists of the combination use of pyrimethamine and sulfadiazine both of which inhibit this activation. Both Pyrimethamine and Sulfadiazine inhibit folic acid synthesis in the parasite with different mechanisms of action and they complement one another to create a synergistic effect. Sulfadiazine works by inhibiting dihydropteroate synthase (DHPS). Pyrimethamine works by inhibiting dihydrofolate reductase enzyme (DHFR), which leads to shortage in tetrahydrofolate (THF). THF is the active form of folic acid, also called vitamin B9. It has a key role in the synthesis of purine and pyrimidine and thus, in the production of DNA-strands during cell replication. Unfortunately, this effect is not specific to the parasite but also interferes with the host's production of active folic acid. A potential adverse effect of this treatment regimen is bone marrow suppression. This suppression may lead to neutropenia, anemia and thrombocytopenia, which are avoidable with simultaneous administration of activated folic acid during treatment. Leucovorin, an active folic acid, is used to prevent the bone marrow suppression and is recommended to be given concurrently with pyrimethamine and sulfadiazine. Acute toxicity of pyrimethamine consists of neurological (hyperexcitability, convulsions) and gastrointestinal (vomiting, anorexia) symptoms. In extreme situations, respiratory and hemodynamic failure may occur.

The kinetics of the medications are varied in children and some believe that blood levels of the drugs, particularly pyrimethamine should be monitored closely. It is unclear what causes the toxicity from the pyrimethamine. Studies of cancer chemotherapy medication methotrexate which appears also to have its effect through interfering with folic acid activation reveals elevation in homocysteine concentrations in children treated with methotrexate (MTX) for leukemia. The elevation in homocysteine appears to produce an increase in nitric oxide synthesis and vascular disease. It is also found that the elevation of homocysteine concentration results in changes in concentrations of various neurotransmitters. The increased neurotransmitter concentration may be the cause of the hyper-excitability of the baby's nervous system and the seizures.

A study of children that received MTX had significant elevations in adenosine in their cerebrospinal fluid and, when symptomatic, methylxanthines, adenosine receptor antagonists, mitigate the symptoms. Excess homocysteine can be metabolized to sulfur-containing excitatory amino acid neurotransmitters which are agonists of n-methyl D-aspartate (NMDA) receptors which may be involved in the generation of seizures.

There are few studies of the compliance with medication in toxoplasmosis therapy. One study revealed that almost 15% of those placed on these medications either discontinued the drugs or changed the dose because of toxicity or side effects.

Getting back to baby boy V, it was late in the afternoon a few days before Christmas. Information specialist Ashish Bhatnagar was on duty. Ashish was a physician trained in India who was working as a poison information specialist at the poison center. He came into my office with a question about a call he had just taken. A pediatrician called from her office about a five-month-old patient of hers with congenital toxoplasmosis. The child had been treated with pyrimethamine and trimethoprim sulfur since his birth. She said the child developed seizures that weekend and was admitted to a teaching hospital, and they believed the seizures might be related to medication. The physician wanted to confirm this possibility and was asking to speak to a supervisor. I explained that I had very little personal experience with either treating this disease or using this medication, but that I would look into the matter and see what I could find. I did a quick search of the literature to find out if there had been case reports of infants convulsing from pyrimethamine and if there was a way to test for blood levels of the medication. As a faculty member of Rutgers University, I had access, electronically, to a vast system of libraries which enabled me to view articles appearing in tens of thousands of journals. Searching this database for convulsions and pyrimethamine, I was able to find an article, in French, concerning an infant who inadvertently received 100 mg per kilogram of the medication, rather than the prescribed dose of 1 mg per kilogram per day and convulsed. I could not find any references to convulsions occurring from the use of this medication with appropriate dosing. This was one of the very few times that the three years of high school and one year of college French that I struggled through, came in handy. I still remember how to read French, at least scientific French. That article cited some other articles, also in French, that were not immediately available online. I discovered in my reading, that there is no commercially available pediatric dosage formulation for the medication. I searched the internet and found that there was a laboratory that had pyrimethamine levels listed in its catalogue of available tests. As it happened, the chief forensic technologist at that laboratory was someone that I had worked with on previous cases of other toxin-related diseases. I felt comfortable in being able to state that blood levels were available. I called the physician back and discussed the possibility that the pyrimethamine was related to the convulsion and that there was a laboratory that could do blood levels to determine if there had been an overdose. I wondered aloud to the physician if there might have been a problem with the dispensed medication either by the pharmacist who prepared it or in the way the mother administered it. Speaking to the pediatrician I discovered that an old friend of mine was the pediatric infectious disease specialist involved in the care of this patient.

Later that afternoon, checking my emails, I found an email from the pediatric infectious disease physician:

Steve,
   May I run this case briefly with you?

I have been following up an infant for congenital toxoplasmosis—presented at birth as neonatal thrombocytopenic purpura—work-up Toxoplasma IgM and IgG confirmed twice including at Palo Alto. After discussion with an expert on toxoplasmosis we started him on pyrimethamine, Sulfadiazine and leocovorin—doses as recommended. He has been doing very well until he developed a seizure this past week—ended up in PICU [pediatric intensive care unit]—*where after the dose of pyrimethamine, child seized and mother told the family that this is what happened the first time. The hospital's peds neurology is convinced that this is due to Pyrimethamine. I told them to send a level.*

In LexiComp—Pyrimethamine has no CNS [central nervous system] *ADR* [adverse drug reaction] *but sulfadiazine has CNS ADR—one of them is convulsion.*

Have you come across Pyrimethamine toxicity and if so it is dose dependent or idiosyncratic?

I then replied via email to the infectious disease physician:

Funny that you should ask! The PMD called this afternoon. My theory, although PMD says no, is that they got a new Rx and that med was made incorrectly. There is an article in the French literature of a med error resulting in convulsion from a 100X error. I will send it to you tomorrow. It also could be that the suspension was not thoroughly shaken and for months the child received only diluent, then as got down lower in the bottle, got pure drug and thus OD.

A laboratory does quantitative analysis and they can send blood there.

It is amazing that they called you and didn't bother calling us.

The physician replied shortly after receiving my email:

When the hospital called me (I believed it was yesterday morning)—I could not believe it since he has had no problems with it. "Pyrimethamine toxicity?—I recommended to them to send a level. Their peds pharm said levels are not done. I recommended to the PICU resident who was on—there are two sources I can think of to call about levels—Poison Center [this I also told the PMD] *and their chemistry lab. My best bet is NJPIES-Poison Center.*

I called them this morning and they said that they were able to send blood for levels to a lab (?). They are holding off on the Pyrimethamine. So now this child is only on sulfadiazine and leucovorin. I have to come up with an alternate so I left a message with Dr. R who is one of the authors of the chapter on Toxoplasmosis in Feigin and Cherry Textbook of Peds Infectious Diseases.

Your theory is highly plausible since this has to be a compounded drug. How can we prove this?

Looking forward to the article.

My response was that we needed to obtain the bottle of medication which was used by the mother and have it analyzed. I agreed to reach out to the technologist that I knew at the reference laboratory to inquire if her laboratory could analyze the preparation.

It appeared to me that there was some difficulty in communication between the treatment team and the prior treating physicians. This sort of situation was uncommon when I was a resident in training; the pediatricians in practice were then true primary care providers for children. During residency we were taught about the importance of continuity of care and were encouraged to follow patients longitudinally. When a patient was hospitalized, the primary care pediatrician, who really knew the patient and patient's family best, would make rounds every day in the hospital early in the morning and see his or her patients. This activity has virtually ceased in the modern era of medicine as practiced today. In the current practice, patient care is provided by a "hospitalist," usually a full-time hospital employee, or a group, who care for the patients while the patients are in the hospital, sometimes with residents and sometimes without. The hospitalists work "shifts" so that not only is there lack of continuity with the primary care physician, but there is often three or more different physicians in a day. With the current system, the pediatrician in the office has no responsibility for the care of a patient while the patient is in the hospital. If the pediatrician cares to visit, it is done on a non-medical management procedure. In this case, the child's attending physician and the previous pediatric infectious disease physician depended upon telephone communication with the hospital to try to ascertain what was happening. The apparent problem with the preparation was not well appreciated by the in-hospital treatment team which had little knowledge of the continuity of care of the child.

In thinking about the possibility of pyrimethamine-associated seizures, I considered that there could be two possibilities responsible. Since the medication was compounded by a local pharmacy which had no previous experience with the medication, and since it was made as a suspension, the preparation could be at fault, rather than a mother's error in dispensing it. I considered the possibility that the pharmacist, not used to compounding this medication, might have made a dilutional error resulting in a super high concentration of the medication in the suspension. Additionally, suspensions require significant shaking to ensure equal dispersion of medication throughout the bottle. It is similar to shaking a bottle of salad oil which sediments back down before you have the chance to pour it onto your salad leaving most of the top layer without spices.

That analogy is to a medication bottle from which, during the early part of its use, the child may be getting only the supernatant (liquid diluent) for the drug and not the real drug. In time, as the administration of medication from that bottle continued, the diluent would be pretty much gone leaving almost pure drug. At that point, the child would get a much higher concentration of the drug, which could cause the seizures.

Later, I called the private doctor and spoke to her about my theory. The thought of the mother being unable to mix the suspension properly jumped to the top of the theories. I discussed the French report of a child who presented with convulsions after receiving medication which was 100 times more concentrated than it was supposed to be. I agreed to send a copy of the article to her and to the infectious disease consultant. I contacted a technologist that I had worked with on another issue who worked for NMS Laboratories, one of the best known forensic laboratories in the country. I wanted to determine if they could do a quantitative analysis of both the blood as well as the medication itself. I was told that yes, they could help us pin down both the child's blood levels and the concentration of the compounded medication.

When I again spoke to the infectious disease specialist later in the day, I learned that the family was in need of a new bottle of pyrimethamine so the pediatrician did write a new prescription. The revelation that a new prescription had preceded the events altered my theory about the lack of proper mixing and raised the possibility of incorrect preparation of the medication itself.

Clarifying the situation with the pediatrician, she stated that two days prior to the presentation to the Emergency Department, the mother called her stating that she was running out of medication. The pediatrician called the pharmacy and gave a verbal order for the medication to be dispensed incorporating an increase in the dose to account for the child's weight. The following day the child was seen in the pediatrician's office for follow-up. The mother was a bit confused about the new dose, so the physician gave instructions on the use of medication dispensing syringes. She gave the mother two syringes to use, placing a mark on the syringe to denote the exact dose she wanted the mother to administer. This caused me to think of another possible theory for an overdose occurring. Years before this case, we were called in consultation about a woman with Alzheimer's who was prescribed medication in patch form. The instructions which came with the patches showed possible locations for the patch to be placed, but did not clearly indicate only one patch at a time. The woman ended up in an Emergency Department with nine patches on her. Perhaps giving the mother two syringes and telling her how much of each syringe she was to give confused her into giving two syringes full of medication. According to the pediatrician's recollection of the story, the following day the mother noticed that the child was acting strangely, was crying more than usual and was very difficult to console. The mother thought the child was having jerky motions of his upper and lower extremities when laying down. She stated that the child also had some vomiting. Because of these strange observations, the mother took the patient to a local Emergency Department. The staff in the hospital Emergency Room felt that the child was teething and he was sent home. Later in the course of the child's illness, I reached out to the medical director of the emergency department at that hospital and, in a review of the emergency room record, there was no mention of the history of congenital toxoplasmosis, no discussion about the medication the child was receiving and no suggestion to stop administering it to the child.

The following day he was given his medication as scheduled. He again started acting strange, so the mother took him to the pediatrician's office. In the pediatrician's office the child was noted to have an episode of vomiting and a generalized tonic clonic seizure. Emergency Medical Services (EMS, aka ambulance) was called. Upon arrival EMS noted the seizure activity. The patient was given anti-seizure medication, lorazepam, and was transported to the emergency department of a tertiary care facility. He was noted on arrival in the emergency room to be actively seizing. The seizures terminated with the use of a combination of the anti-seizure medicine lorazepam and fosphenytoin. He was also given a dose of antibiotics for a possible covert infection. Meningitis is always a consideration when an infant suffers a convulsion. He was admitted to the pediatric intensive care unit.

An evaluation for possible infection was performed. All of the cultures eventually returned as negative. A repeat MRI of the brain was also reported as negative on the day of the hospitalization. The patient was not given any pyrimethamine or sulfadiazine on the initial day. The next day it was decided to start the child back on his medications so that there would be no chance that the toxoplasmosis would flare up in the hospital. The hospital pharmacy did not carry pyrimethamine so they used the patient's own home supply on the following day of hospitalization. About thirty minutes after receiving a dose of the home medication the patient experienced a seizure consisting of his eyes gazing up and rolling of his head, then the seizure progressed down to include his entire body. The seizure resolved after the administration of lorazepam.

Due to the timing of the seizure in relation to the administration of the medication, the decision was made to discontinue the pyrimethamine but continue the sulfadiazine. When I was called and told about what happened, I suggested to the hospital that the bottle of the pyrimethamine be sent to me and that I would have it assayed to determine the concentration. The patient was observed in the hospital and had no further episodes of seizures. The hospital had some blood samples available from earlier in the hospitalization and a blood concentrations of pyrimethamine was drawn on day eight. The blood samples were sent with the medication bottle to the reference lab.

The pyrimethamine concentrations returned after the child had been discharged from the hospital. The first level drawn about eighteen hours into the admission was 3.8 mcg/mL which is almost ten times the usual upper-limit of the therapeutic dose. The second level four days after stopping the medication was 1.2 µg. A third level obtained eleven days after stopping the pyrimethamine was undetectable. The results of the analysis of the dispensed medication revealed a concentration of 94 mg/mL, rather than the prescribed 2 mg/mL.

The picture we can recreate in this case is one that I term a "perfect storm." The treating physicians were faced with an unusual disease, one which a single physician may never see during his or her career. The medication used to treat it is an unusual one, again one that the physicians would not be accustomed to ordering. The medication does not come in a pediatric preparation, so an adult formulation has to be adapted to a form that can be administered to a child. That combined to become the perfect storm, further complicated by the hospital's assumption that the preparation was not to blame. Physicians faced with an unusual situation need to muster all of their efforts to prevent error, or this outcome will recur.

Suggested Reading

Elmalem J, Poulet B, Garnier R, et al. Les accidents graves lors de la prescription de pyrimethamine chez les nourrissons traits pour une toxoplasmose. Therapie. 1985;40:357–9.

Genuine M, Freihuber C, Girard L, et al. Intoxication neonatale a la pyrimethamine: un risqué lie a l'absence de forme galenique pediatrique? Arch Pediatr. 2011;18:1084–6.

Robert-Gangneux F. It is not only the cat that did it: how to prevent and treat congenital toxoplasmosis. J Infect. 2014;68:5125–33.

Index

© Springer International Publishing AG 2017
S.M. Marcus, *Medical Toxicology: Antidotes and Anecdotes*,
DOI 10.1007/978-3-319-51029-3